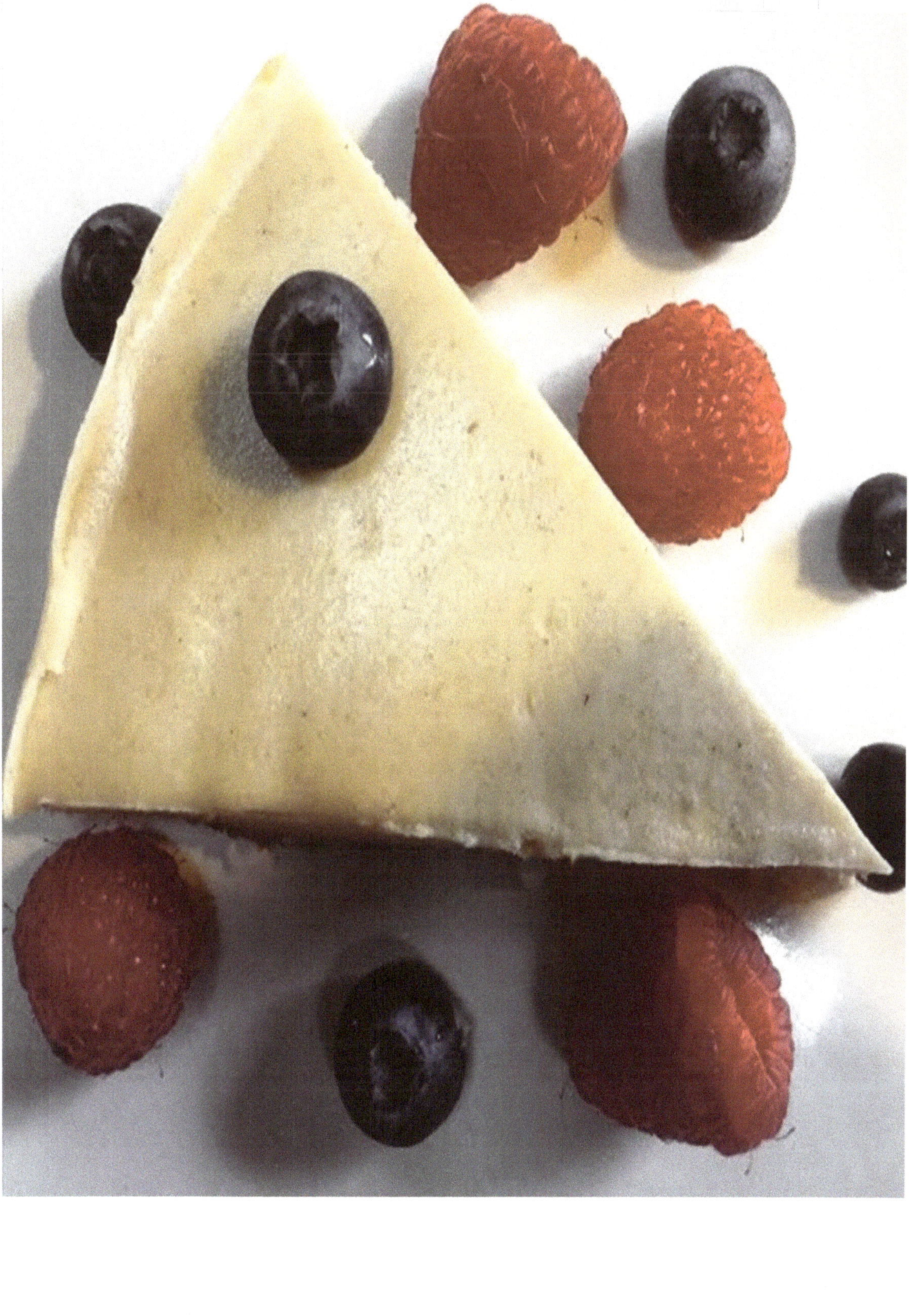

eat! easy everyday raw vegan recipes! by K.L. Strayhorn

© 2016 by Align Your Health® Publishing House. All rights reserved.

No part of this book may be reproduced in any form written, electronic, recording, or photocopying without written permission of the publisher or author. Books may be purchased in bulk quantity and/or special sales by contacting the publisher, Align Your Health® Publishing House, at 5 Awbury Road, Philadelphia, Pennsylvania 19138 or by email at info@ayhlife.com.

Publisher: Align Your Health® Publishing House, a division of SYSWC Marketing and Business Development, Inc.

Editor: John R. Winters Jr.

Photography/Illustration: TableTop™ Photography, Inc.

Cover Design: SYSWC Marketing and Business Development, Inc. and TableTop™ Photography, Inc.

Interior Design: SYSWC Marketing and Business Development, Inc.

Library of Congress Catalog Number: 2015921341
ISBN: 978-0-9971634-0-7
eBook ISBN: 978-0-9971634-1-4
Includes Index
First Edition

Copyright © 2016 by Align Your Health® Publishing House.
All rights reserved, including the right to reproduce this book, and/or its contents, or portions thereof in any form.

Printed in the United States of America

SYSWC Marketing and Business Development, Inc.
Align Your Health® Publishing House
5 Awbury Road
Philadelphia, Pennsylvania 19138
www.ayhlife.com

A Note of Gratitude

There are so many beautiful souls that have shared with me their wisdom, light, and love on my journey thus far. These energies have sustained me during my lowest lows and highest highs.
For that, I will be forever grateful.

Kathryn Hill Strayhorn (Mommy)

Lloyd Strayhorn (Daddy)

John R. Winters Jr.

Rahsaan, Amaar, Llonice, Darrien Jaleel (DJ), and Kiana

all of my beautiful nieces and nephews, my extended family, dear friends,

and Beverly

Thank You!

Contents

Preface, I

Everyday Pantry Essentials, II

My Journey to Raw, 1

A Little Bit of Q & A, 3

Beverages, 7

Breakfast, 19

Desserts, 31

Dips, Sauces, Spreads, 53

Entrees, 69

Sides, 85

Soups & Salads, 101

Raw Vegan Glossary, 113

Soaking & Sprouting Guide, 119

Index, 121

Preface

Dearest Readers,

Soon after we take our first breath of life, we eat. That sacred and special time at the beginning of our human existence is spent with us being nourished in the simplest, yet most loving way.

eat! easy everyday raw vegan recipes! is a book designed to give its readers a simple approach to nourishing the body. As adults, we tend to become completely separated from what the body *needs* and what we *want*. Many of us *want* to have "wash board abs" or *want* to look perfect in a pair of jeans. And if the pursuit of those goals are done in a holistic and self-loving way, then great. However, most times that is not the case. We lose ourselves in the striving and search for solace in ways completely unrelated to nourishing the body and ultimately feeding the soul.

eat! encourages you to do just that, nourish your body and feed your soul. The recipes are simple, easy to follow, and provide the groundwork for you to explore nutritious, fun, and delicious raw vegan recipes. The recipes in *eat!* will help you to establish a foundation for your journey towards a healthier lifestyle and more complex raw vegan recipes.

Enjoy this book with love and happily *eat!*

Kindly & in good health always,

Keirra

December, 2015

Everyday Pantry Essentials

The recipes in *eat!* have been lovingly created using the following everyday pantry essentials. Take this essentials list with you to the grocery store!

Oils (recipes in *eat!* utilize ONLY these oils):

Organic Cold-pressed (expeller pressed) Extra Virgin Olive Oil
Organic Cold-pressed (expeller pressed) Coconut Oil
Organic Cold-pressed (expeller pressed) Sesame Oil

Sea Salt (recipes in *eat!* utilize ONLY coarse ground sea salt):

Celtic Sea Salt
*Himalayan Salt is also an option.

Sweeteners (a great date paste sweetener alternative is inside the book!):

Raw Date Sugar (dehydrated and ground whole dates)
Raw Agave
Maple Syrup, Grade B

Nuts & Seeds (make sure the nuts are raw and unsalted):

Unpasteurized Raw Almonds (usually sourced from Italy/Spain)
Raw Hazelnuts
Raw Hemp Seeds
Raw Macadamia Nuts
Raw Pecans
Raw Sesame Seeds
Raw Walnuts

Herbs & Spices (fresh herbs and spices can also be used):

Dried Basil
Cayenne Pepper
Cumin
Dried Oregano
Onion Powder
Dried Sage
Dried Thyme

Sea Veggies (check your local markets or online for these products):

Nori/Dulse
Wakame
Kelp Granules/Powder
Sea Moss (whole or powder)

Miscellaneous (great to have on hand):

Jicama
Raw Apple Cider Vinegar
Young Thai Coconut

My Journey to Raw

Before sharing how I found myself living this amazing and wonderful raw vegan lifestyle, I should go back to where my vegan journey began.

Growing up, I faced many challenges with self-esteem. By the time I graduated from college I had no real positive self-perception and my greatest desire was to transform my low self-esteem into one of self-love, acceptance, and appreciation. I was not sure how this transformation was going to occur, but I was sure that I was committed to fulfilling my deepest desire, which was to know, unequivocally, self-love.

Our greatest desires, whether we acknowledge them or not, reside in the deepest parts of our heart and soul. To reach this place of depth, I veered towards health and wellness, taking yoga classes and saying farewell to fast food and soda. At that time, nearly fifteen years ago, I did not even know the word 'vegan' existed let alone what it meant. I simply went in the direction of practices that, for me, felt supportive, nurturing, and honestly, practical for embarking on the journey of knowing self-love. Making gradual and slow changes allowed me the time and space to fully process what I was doing and, more importantly, why. Many times, we hop from one trendy diet to another not fully understanding what is driving us to starve ourselves, exercise excessively, and participate in a slew of other unhealthy practices that will only, at best, provide an exterior change.

My soul wanted more, so I followed its curiosity with a willingness to learn and experience the unknown and achieve my greatest good. My mom would always say, "Whatever you are looking for, the universe will bring to you." Such a simple and profound sentiment turned out to be quite true. Shortly after I fully committed to my personal journey of discovering self-love, I met my husband John. John had tapped in to New York City's vegan community. Luckily for me, many of our date nights consisted of eating the most delicious vegan food at some of the best vegan restaurants in New York City. What I could not get over was how tasty this vegan food was and at the same time, better for your health. It was a total win-win. For an entire year, John and I dated and it seemed like all we did was happily **eat!**

Upon our one year anniversary, I had transitioned to a fully vegan diet! Who knew that a romance could change your health, not just your heart. I will forever be grateful for this time in my life and the foundation it laid for me to fulfill on my journey of self-love and acceptance. Fortifying my health with a plant-based (vegan) diet and yoga was pivotal in building my self-esteem. Not only was it good for my physical and mental health, it also became a great creative outlet. I found so much joy in the challenge of preparing vegan foods and coming up with new dishes that were satisfying and healthy. Recreating SAD (Standard American Diet) dishes by making them vegan was of particular interest to me while building my culinary repertoire. I started thinking of it as "vegan-izing" recipes. A little over ten years later, I have carried this same curiosity, joy, and enthusiasm into preparing raw vegan dishes that are familiar, accessible, simple, and delicious.

Transitioning from vegan to raw vegan was another fated experience. Being the owner of a yoga studio and wellness center, business-wise, life had taken its toll. While yoga is truly one of the most widely known modalities for stress relief, business ownership is its complete opposite. Business owners tend to work non-stop hours building their company to get it off the ground. I was admittedly over-worked and not taking time to replenish the creative and energetic channels that I used to develop a successful yoga studio. Feeling depleted, I found myself again looking for a reprieve. And true to my mom's sentiment, the universe brought to me a soul-stirring look at *raw* plant-based (vegan) food. I wound up meeting a woman, Beverly, who had a raw vegan diet for over three decades.

Beverly's sharing with me, her wisdom and honesty about food, the heart, the self/soul, and how they are all very much connected, was another experience in my life that was transformative. Again, I found myself completely in gratitude and honestly honored for what the universe had brought to me as what I can only describe as a gift.

This book is my way of sharing the gifts of food wisdom that was bestowed upon me in my times of need. I truly hope this book is brought to you when you need it most! Let it inspire you to become your best self, reach for your greatest good, love fully, and **eat!**

A little Bit of Q & A
with the author

1. **What do you mean by "live foods?" Does it move or something?**

Live food or living food is food that has not had its natural enzymes destroyed or "killed" through the process of cooking. Live or living food is not heated above 115° Fahrenheit (46° Celsius), thereby maintaining its nutrient structure.

2. **Is there a difference between vegan, vegetarian and/or other meatless diets?**

Yes! Alkaline Raw Vegan is a plant-based diet in which only non-hybrid, non-GMO (genetically modified organism), non-soy, non-wheat, low starch foods are consumed. An alkaline raw vegan diet consists primarily of leafy greens, fruits, vegetables, nuts, seeds, and herbs.

A vegan diet includes only plant-based foods. No dairy (milk, eggs, cheese) or meat (beef, pork, chicken, turkey, or fish) are consumed.

Vegetarian is a diet in which one does not consume any meat, but may eat dairy products.

Pescatarian is a diet category in which a person does not eat meat (beef, pork, chicken, or turkey) but does eat sea food.

An omnivore diet includes consuming both plants and animals.

3. **Which kind of diet do you see yourself as having? Or do you prefer to not be labeled?**

To be most accurate, I do eat a primarily alkaline raw vegan diet, however, occasionally I may eat sprouted, cooked quinoa.

4. How does one get started with a raw vegan diet?

As with life in general, we all have different "starting points," be they socially, economically, physically, etc. So keeping this in mind, be patient and kind to yourself upon the first thought of adopting a raw vegan diet. Also, remember to be curious, willing to learn, and have fun! Don't stop eating (unless you are intentionally fasting) or your body will "freak out" and possibly undermine your new journey towards a more conscientious diet.

5. Where is the best place to shop for raw plant-based (vegan) ingredients?

Grocery stores, local markets, or supermarkets in most communities will carry raw/live fruits and vegetables (produce). Basic produce such as apples, oranges, bananas, leafy greens, broccoli, tomatoes, onions, etc. can be found in these markets. Finding specialty (less common) items such as sea vegetables, Italian raw almonds, burdock root, bladderwrack, etc. may take a small amount of investigative work. Visit the international markets or community co-op's in your city or town. Also, utilizing the internet can be of great benefit for tracking down specialty items.

6. Are there special pots, pans, or utensils used to make these dishes?

Yes and no. You can use most of the kitchen utensils that you already have to get started with a raw vegan diet. The same prep knife, cutting board, blender, and mixing bowl will work just fine for most dishes. However, a dehydrator, a high-power blender, and a juicer will absolutely come in handy and make preparing raw vegan dishes much more easy and fun!

7. Are these dishes a budget buster or does it save money?

Again, yes and no. Most diners know that when eating out at a restaurant the cost of a steak is typically more expensive than a garden salad. Taking this same approach, adopting a plant-based diet could be a money saver depending on your prior food spending habits. Conversely, if the popular dollar menu or all you can eat establishments is where you were spending your food dollars then yes, a raw vegan diet may seem like a budget buster. It's really all relative to your spending habits.

8. Does one have to develop a taste for live foods?

It honestly depends on the raw vegan dish/dessert. Also, consider that after years of eating the SAD (Standard American Diet) way, most times, taste buds have "tuned-out" the natural taste of food. It has almost become white noise in the background to the symphony of flavors that raw vegan food provides. With that being said, take eating a raw plant-based diet as an opportunity to experiment, challenge yourself, and have fun finding flavors that make your palate sing.

9. Does it take long to prepare these dishes?

Preparing raw vegan dishes usually does not take any longer than preparing any other kind of meal and can sometimes be faster than preparing a SAD meal. The one caveat is that depending on which raw vegan dish you decide to prepare, the wait time can be considerable. Again, take this on as a fun, exploratory challenge.

10. Do live food dishes have a shelf-life, or should they be eaten soon after they're prepared?

Fresh is always best. Many people love the smell and taste of freshly baked bread or a fresh pot of coffee in the morning. In theory, the same idea of "fresh is best" would apply. Raw vegan food is best eaten fresh, kept in the refrigerator, or stored in a freezer. Some raw vegan foods, upon being dehydrated, will maintain their freshness up to a point over time.

11. Which dishes are best served cold, hot, or both?

In general, raw vegan desserts are best served cold, and some even frozen, depending on the dessert. Most raw vegan savory items can be warmed in a dehydrator or eaten at room temperature and are delicious.

12. What dishes are best made for breakfast, lunch, and/or dinner?

You can find the answers to that question inside the book!

13. Can you give some examples?

After spending time enjoying and eating raw vegan food, your body's natural intelligence will be in full swing. Let your body tell you what to eat for breakfast or dinner on a particular day. Our lifestyles are full, fun, and busy. On some days we may be okay with just a smoothie for breakfast on other days something a little bit more substantial may work best.

14. What are some of the do's and don'ts to making these dishes?

Do be proud of yourself for trying! Raw vegan is probably not the food you grew up eating. Do be patient when trying these recipes. Do have fun preparing the recipes, and don't quit on your first fail. Say hello to the failure, thank it for showing you where you went wrong, and then DO try again!

15. Are there other suggestions or recommendations regarding live foods?

Be a sponge, read, talk to people who have similar diets, speak with your local grocers, be curious, and be excited. Like a child learning how to ride a bike, absorb the entire experience and have fun!

16. Besides "eat!," would you recommend any other books?

Sure!
- **Numbers & You,** by Lloyd Strayhorn
- **You Can Heal Your Life,** by Louise L. Hay
- **The Yoga Sutras of Pantanjali,** Swami Satchidananda
- **Love Is in the Earth: A Kaleidoscope of Crystals,** by Melody

Having reading materials and tools that will fortify and encourage you spiritually, mentally, and physically on your journey from SAD to raw vegan can be incredibly beneficial! Enjoy the journey - the peaks and the pits, and of course... **eat!**

Beverages

Almond Milk

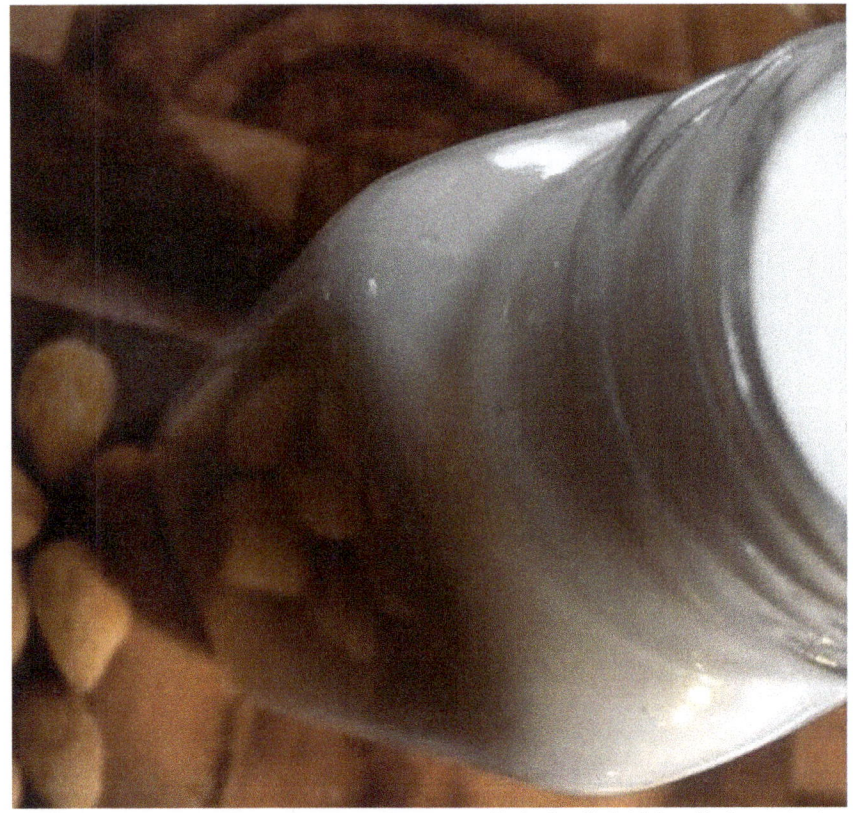

Photo Credit: TableTop Photography, Inc.

INGREDIENTS:

- 3 cups water
- 1 and 1/2 cups soaked almonds (see page 119)

DIRECTIONS:
place ingredients in blender. Blend until completely smooth, strain liquid from blender through a cheesecloth or nut milk bag. Store milk in refrigerator.

HANDY TOOLS:
food processor and cheesecloth/nut milk bag.

eat! easy everyday raw vegan recipes! | 8

Carob Seamoss Shake

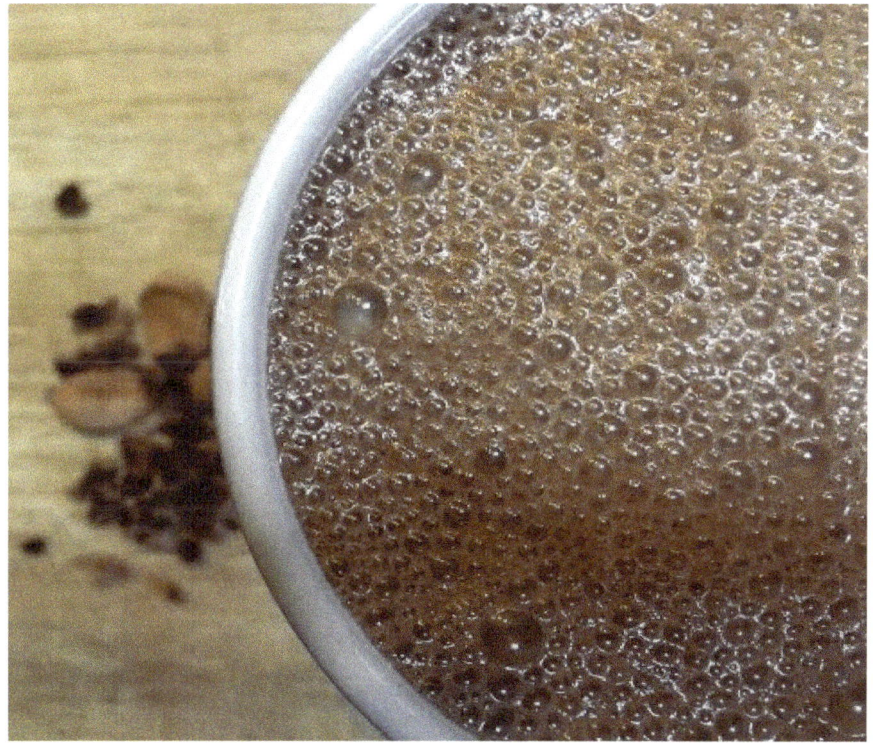

Photo Credit: TableTop Photography, Inc.

INGREDIENTS:

- 2 and 1/2 cups almond milk (see page 8)
- 3 Tbsp raw agave or date paste (see page 43)
- 2 and 1/2 Tbsp raw carob powder
- 1 and 1/2 tsp sea moss (see page 117)

DIRECTIONS:
place all ingredients in blender and blend until well combined. Serve cold or over ice.

HANDY TOOLS:
blender.

Cinnamon Lime Mocktail

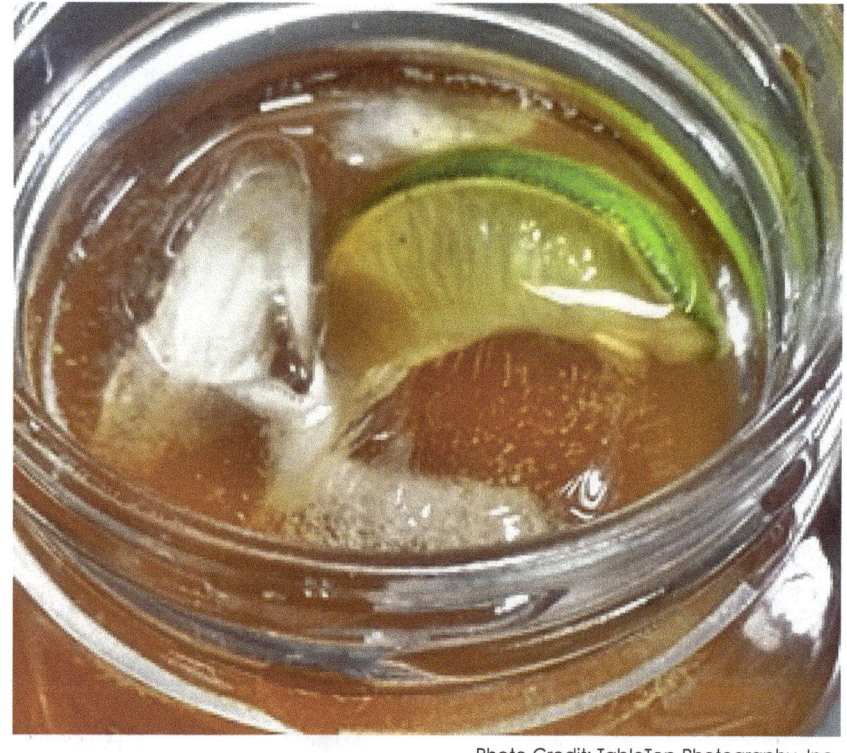

Photo Credit: TableTop Photography, Inc.

INGREDIENTS:

- 4 cups water
- 1/4 cup raw agave or date paste (see page 43)
- 1 Tbsp cinnamon powder
- 1 Tbsp lime juice
- 1 tsp star anise powder
- 1/4 tsp clove powder (optional)

DIRECTIONS:
place all ingredients together in a blender and blend until well combined.

HANDY TOOLS:
blender.

Cinnamon Vanilla Shake

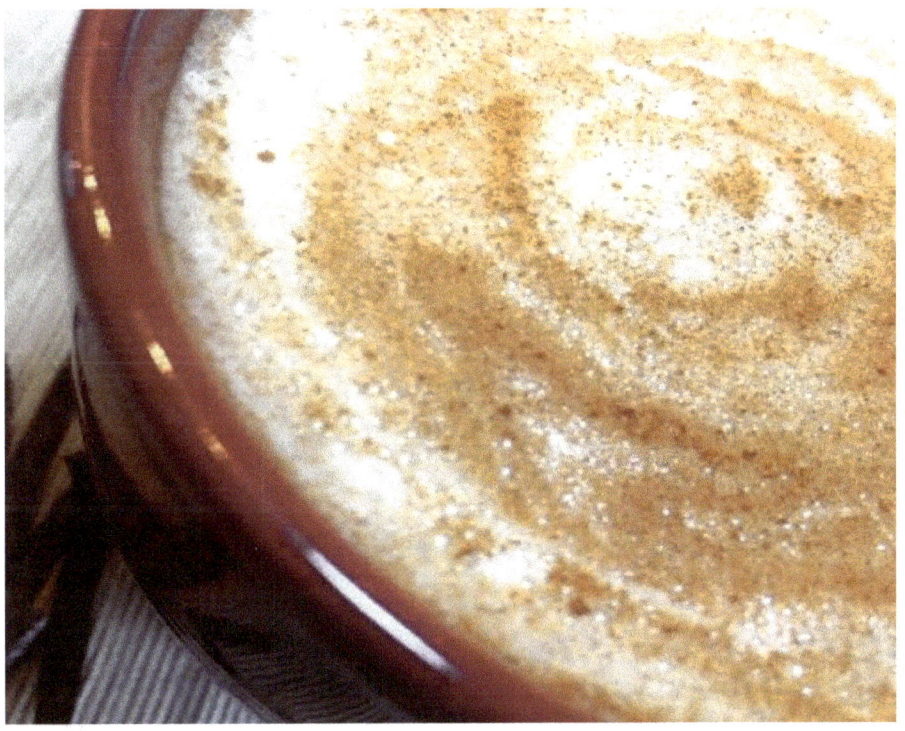

Photo Credit: TableTop Photography, Inc.

INGREDIENTS:

- 2 cups almond milk (see page 8)
- 1/4 cup raw agave or date paste (see page 43)
- 2 tsp cinnamon
- 1 tsp vanilla bean paste (see page 118)
- 1/4 tsp ground clove

DIRECTIONS: place all ingredients in a blender and blend until completely smooth and combined.

HANDY TOOLS: blender.

eat! easy everyday raw vegan recipes!

Citrus Punch

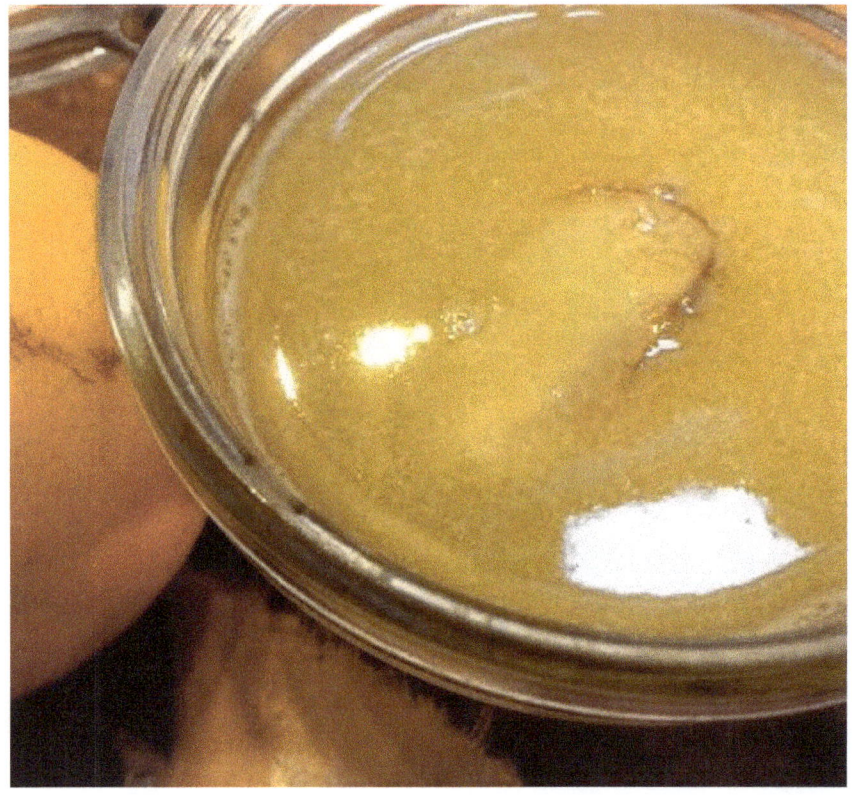

Photo Credit: TableTop Photography, Inc.

INGREDIENTS:

- 2 cups freshly squeezed orange juice
- 1 cup water
- 1 Tbsp lime juice
- 1 Tbsp raw agave or date paste (see page 43)
- 1/4 tsp ginger powder

DIRECTIONS: place ingredients in a blender and blend until well combined.

HANDY TOOLS: blender.

Coconut Milk

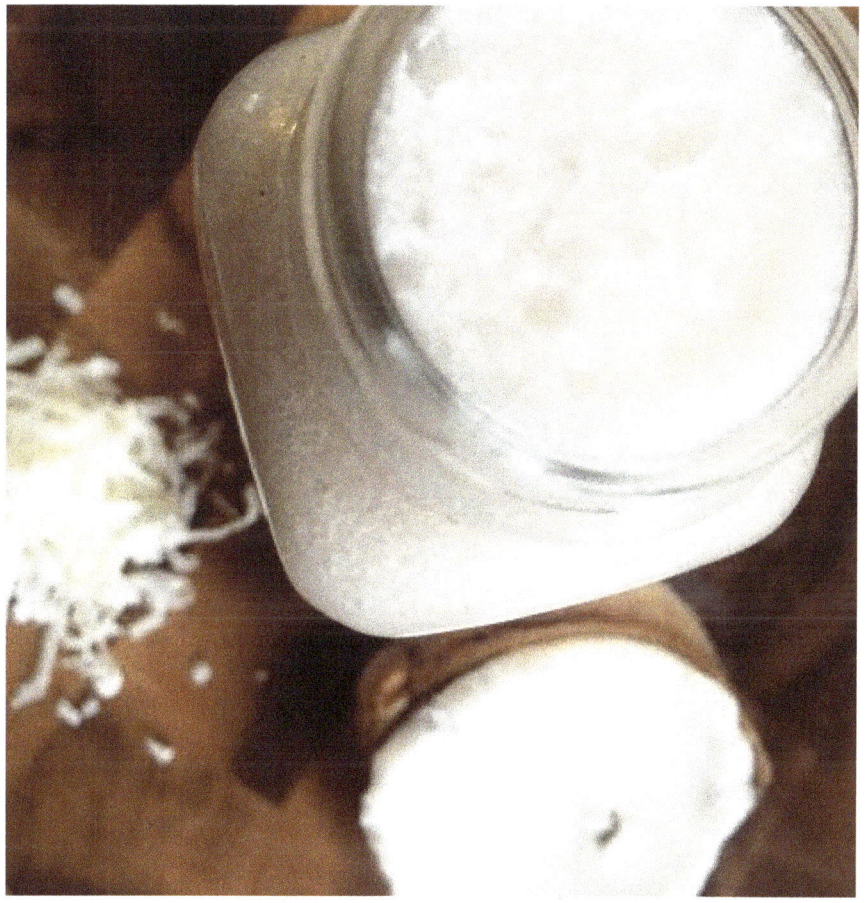

Photo Credit: TableTop Photography, Inc.

INGREDIENTS:

- 1 - 2 young Thai coconuts
- 1 and 1/2 cups fresh coconut water
- 1/2 cup coconut flesh (see page 114)

DIRECTIONS:
open each coconut and drain the water. Pour coconut water into a blender. Scrape out the remaining coconut flesh from each coconut. Place fresh coconut flesh in blender with coconut water and blend until completely smooth.

HANDY TOOLS: blender.

eat! easy everyday raw vegan recipes!

Coconut Chai Milk

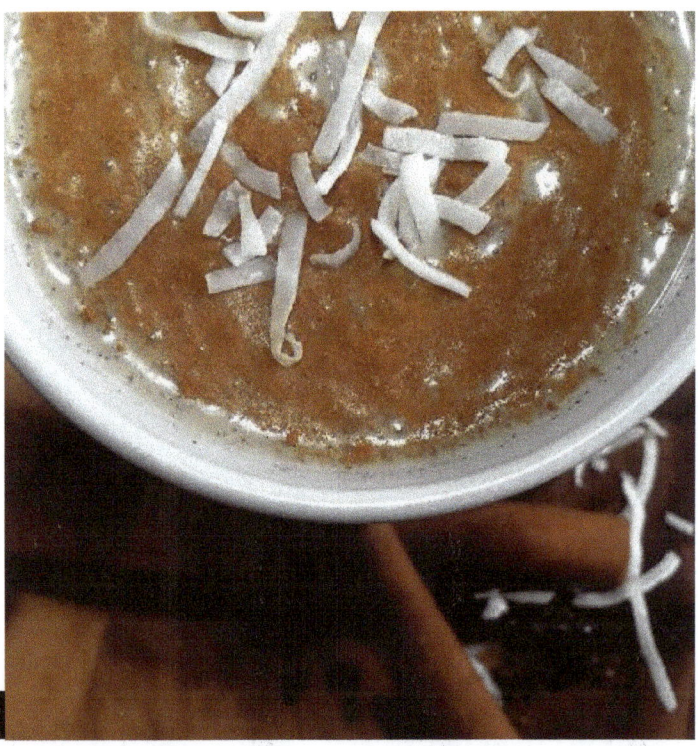

INGREDIENTS:

- 3 cups coconut milk (see page 13)
- 1/3 (packed) cup chopped dates
- 1/2 tsp vanilla bean paste (see page 118)
- 1/2 tsp cinnamon powder
- 1/4 tsp clove powder
- 1/4 tsp ginger powder

Photo Credit: TableTop Photography, Inc.

DIRECTIONS: place all ingredients in blender. Blend until completely smooth.

HANDY TOOLS: food processor.

Papaya Protein Shake

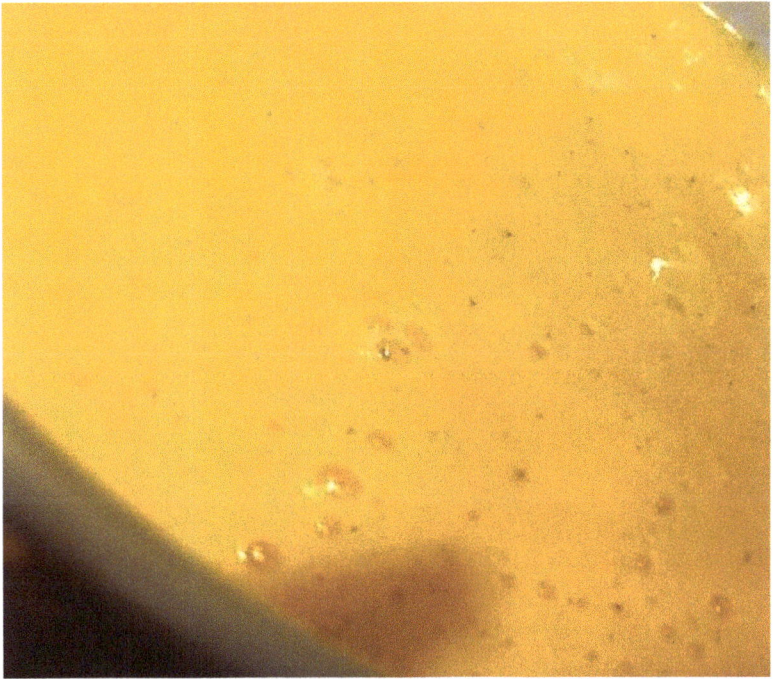

Photo Credit: TableTop Photography, Inc.

INGREDIENTS:

- 1 cup freshly squeezed orange juice
- 1/2 cup chopped papaya
- 1/4 cup sliced baby bananas (see page 113)
- 1/2 Tbsp raw hemp seeds

DIRECTIONS:
place all of the ingredients together in a blender and blend until well combined and completely smooth.

HANDY TOOLS: blender.

Simple Green Goddess Splash

INGREDIENTS:

- 4 cucumbers (preferably Kirby cucumbers)
- 1 cup dandelion leaves
- 1 inch piece fresh ginger

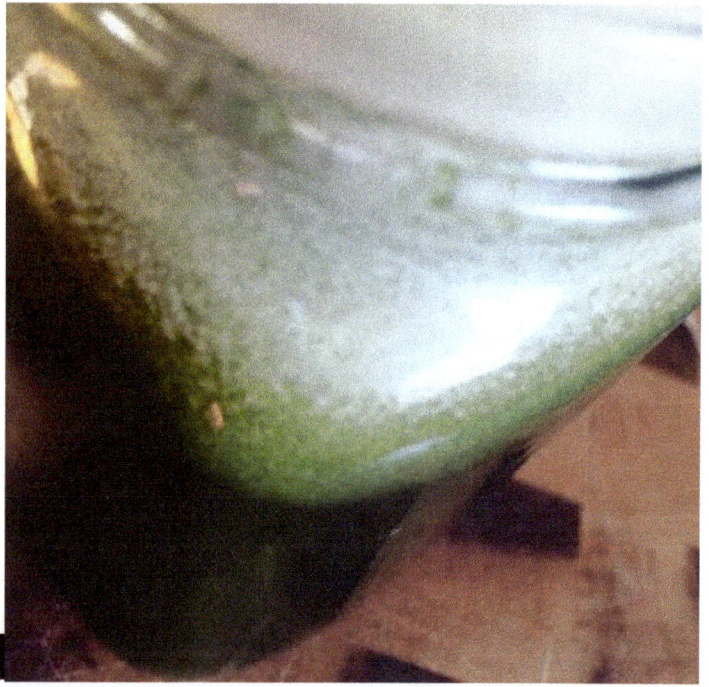

Photo Credit: TableTop Photography, Inc.

DIRECTIONS: chop cucumbers. Press the chopped cucumbers and remaining ingredients through a juicer. Drink immediately.

HANDY TOOLS: juicer.

Watermelon Cooler

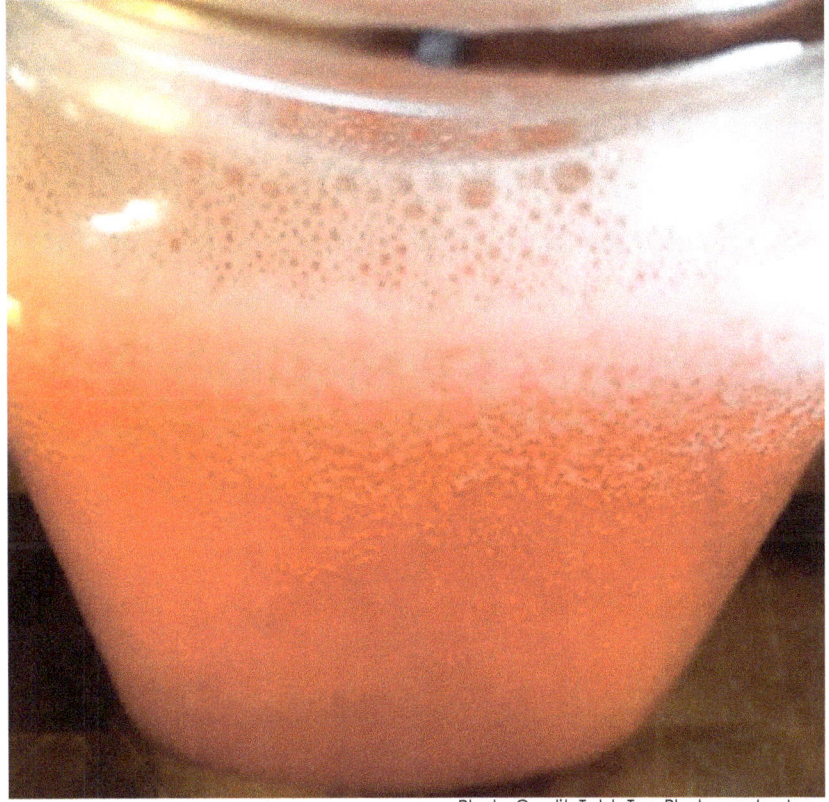

Photo Credit: TableTop Photography, Inc.

INGREDIENTS:

- 4 cups chopped, seeded watermelon (watermelon with seeds)

DIRECTIONS:
place all of the chopped watermelon in a blender and blend until completely smooth. Pour over ice and enjoy.

HANDY TOOLS:
blender.

eat! easy everyday raw vegan recipes!

Breakfast

Apple Cinnamon Granola

INGREDIENTS:

- 1/2 cup chopped sprouted, dehydrated walnuts (see page 117)
- 1/2 cup chopped sprouted, dehydrated pecans (see page 117)
- 1/2 cup chopped apples
- 2 Tbsp raw agave or date paste (see page 43)
- 1/2 tsp cinnamon
- 1/8 tsp Celtic sea salt
- Pinch of clove powder

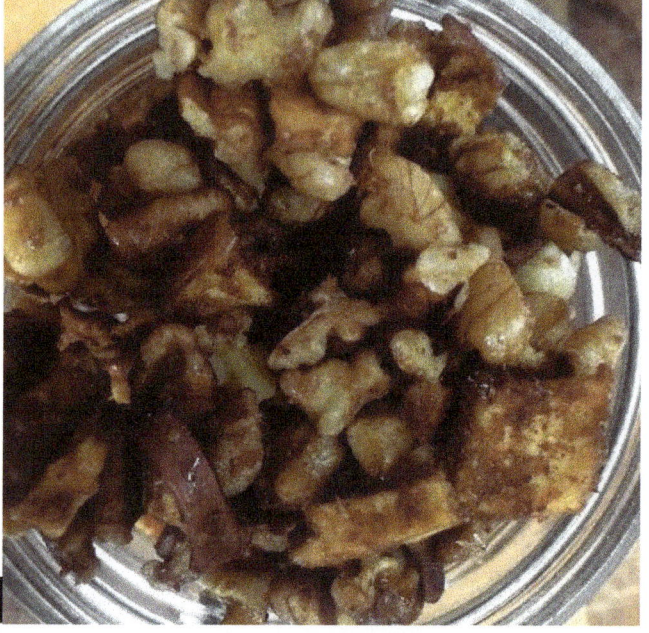

Photo Credit: TableTop Photography, Inc.

DIRECTIONS: place all ingredients together in a medium size bowl and stir until well combined. Place mixture from bowl onto teflex sheet and dehydrate between 95° Fahrenheit (35° Celsius) and 115° Fahrenheit (46° Celsius) for 10 - 12 hours.

HANDY TOOLS: dehydrator and medium size bowl.

Banana Pancakes

INGREDIENTS:

- 2 cups chopped baby bananas
- 1/4 cup raw coconut flour
- 1/2 tsp cinnamon powder (optional)

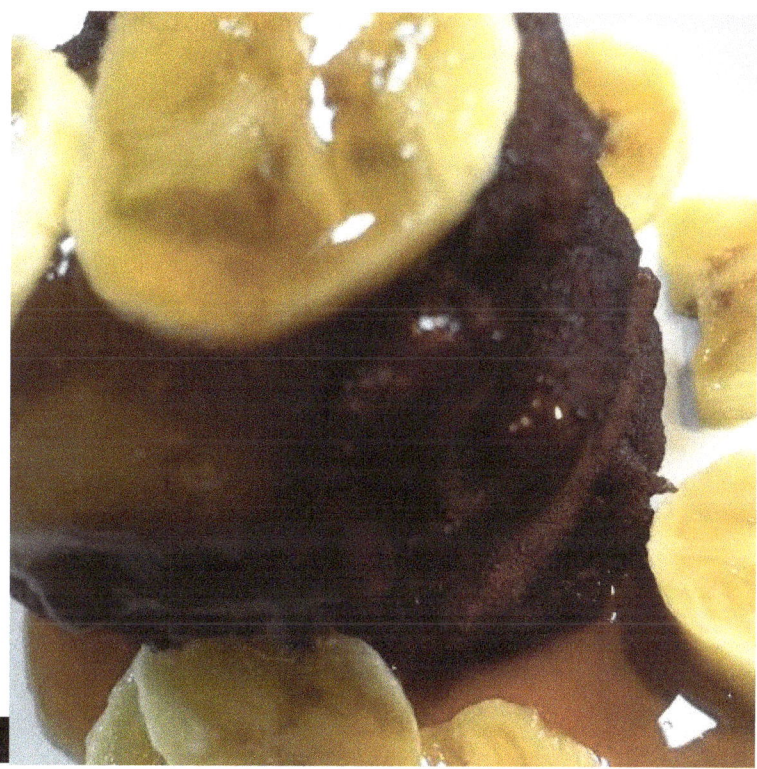

Photo Credit: TableTop Photography, Inc.

DIRECTIONS: place ingredients in blender and blend until completely smooth and creamy. Pour mixture into 3 inch circle pancake shapes on a lightly oiled (with coconut oil) teflex sheet and dehydrate between 95° Fahrenheit (35° Celsius) and 115° Fahrenheit (46° Celsius) for 6 hours, 3 hours on each side.

HANDY TOOLS: dehydrator and blender.

Banana Walnut Oatmeal

INGREDIENTS:

- 1 cup chopped ripe baby bananas
- 1 cup sprouted walnuts (see page 117)
- 1/4 cup chopped apples

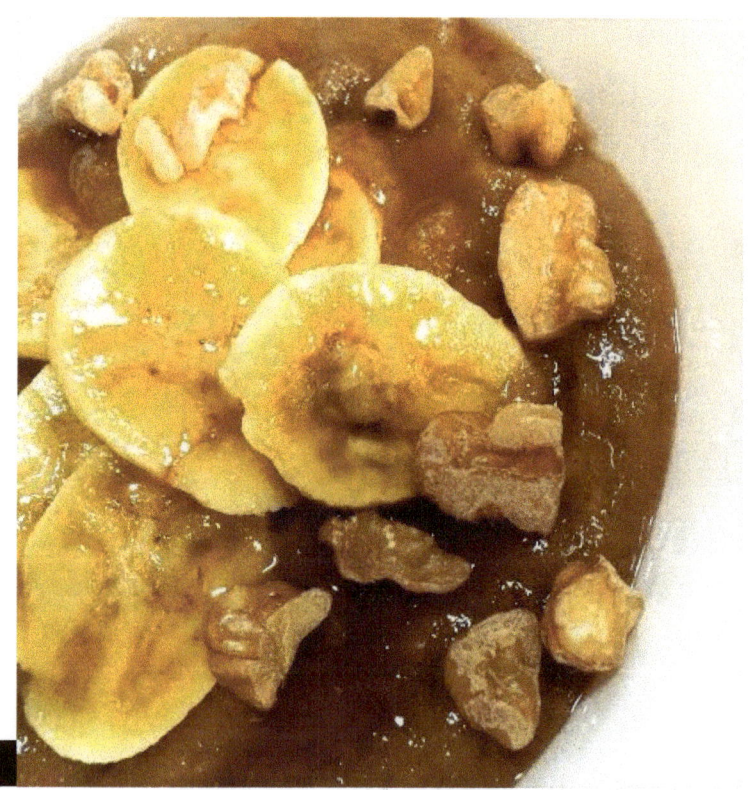

Photo Credit: TableTop Photography, Inc.

DIRECTIONS: place all ingredients in a food processor, blend, leaving the "oatmeal" slightly chunky.

HANDY TOOLS: food processor.

Berry Granola

INGREDIENTS:

- 1/2 cup chopped sprouted, dehydrated walnuts (see page 117)
- 1/2 cup chopped sprouted, dehydrated pecans (see page 117)
- 1/4 cup fresh blueberries
- 2 Tbsp soaked goji berries (soaked for 2 hours)
- 1 Tbsp raw agave or date paste (see page 43)
- 1/8 tsp cinnamon
- 1/8 tsp Celtic sea salt

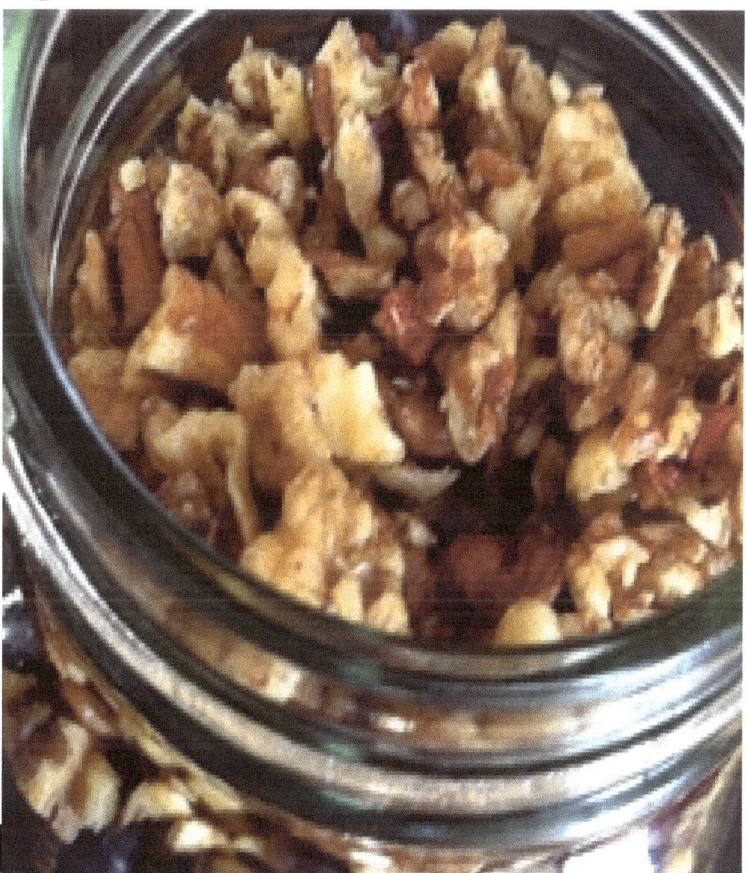

Photo Credit: TableTop Photography, Inc.

DIRECTIONS: place all ingredients together in a medium size bowl and stir until well combined. Place ingredients on a teflex sheet and dehydrate between 95° Fahrenheit (35° Celsius) and 115° Fahrenheit (46° Celsius) for 10 - 12 hours.

HANDY TOOLS: dehydrator and medium size bowl

Breakfast Crepes

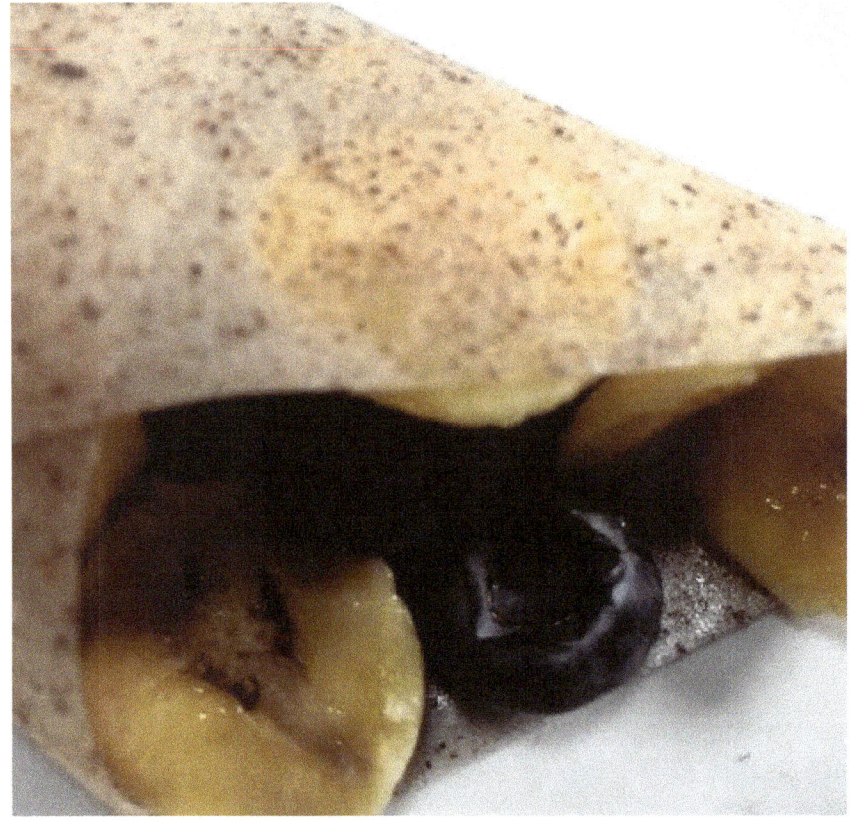

Photo Credit: TableTop Photography, Inc.

INGREDIENTS:

- 1 cup coconut yogurt (see page 29)
- 1/2 cup fresh fruit (blackberries, bananas, etc.)

DIRECTIONS:
spread coconut yogurt on teflex sheet in 6 inch diameter circles and dehydrate between 95º Fahrenheit (35º Celsius) and 115º Fahrenheit (46º Celsius) each side for 4 - 6 hours. Fill with fresh fruit. Optional, drizzle with agave or maple syrup.

HANDY TOOLS: dehydrator.

eat! easy everyday raw vegan recipes!

Breakfast

Smoothie Bowl

INGREDIENTS:

- 1/2 cup freshly squeezed orange juice
- 1/2 cup chopped ripe baby bananas
- 1/2 cup ripe mango (reserve 2 Tbsp for garnish)
- 1/2 cup raspberries
- 1/4 cup avocado
- 1 Tbsp raw hemp seeds (reserve 1 tsp for garnish)
- 1 Tbsp goji berries (reserve 1 tsp for garnish)

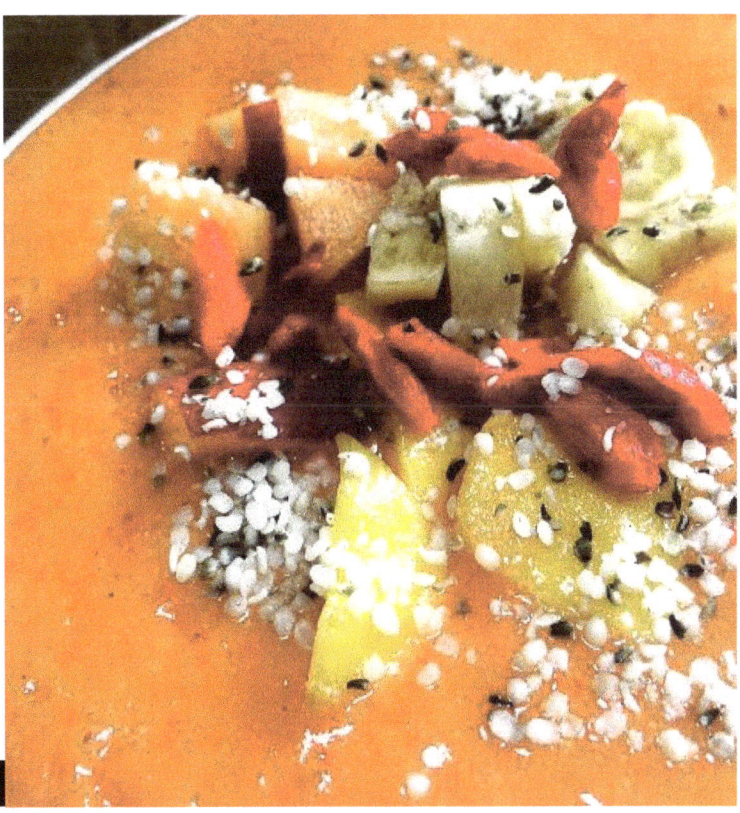

Photo Credit: TableTop Photography, Inc.

DIRECTIONS:
place all of the ingredients (except ingredients reserved for garnish) in a blender and blend until completely smooth. Serve in a bowl. Garnish top with reserved fruit and hemp seeds.

HANDY TOOLS: blender.

Butternut Hash Browns

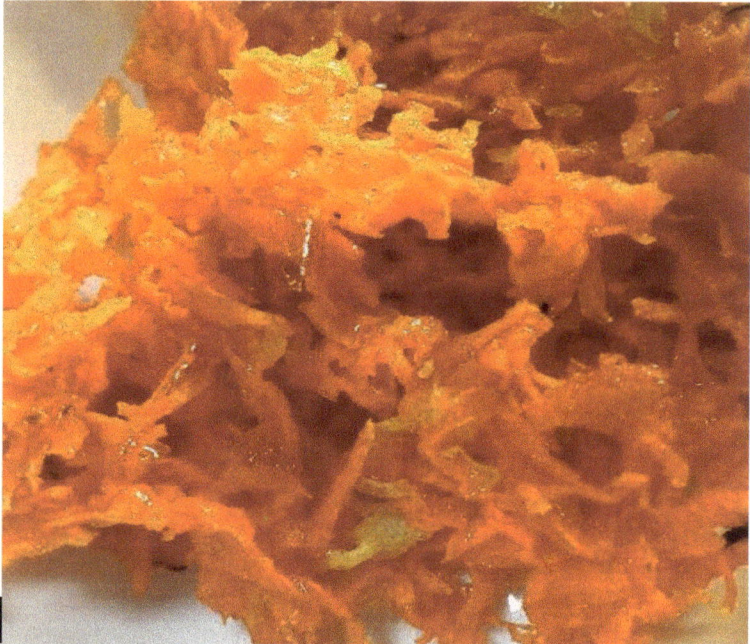

Photo Credit: TableTop Photography, Inc.

INGREDIENTS:

- 2 cups shredded butternut squash
- 1/4 cup chopped yellow onion
- 2 Tbsp olive oil
- 1/2 tsp Celtic sea salt
- 1/8 tsp crushed red pepper flakes (optional)

DIRECTIONS: stir all ingredients together until well combined. Spread on teflex sheet and dehydrate between 95º Fahrenheit (35º Celsius) and 115º Fahrenheit (46º Celsius) for 10 -12 hours.

HANDY TOOLS: grater and dehydrator.

eat! easy everyday raw vegan recipes!

Cinnamon Apple Sauce

INGREDIENTS:

- 1 and 1/2 cup chopped apples
- 1/2 tsp cinnamon

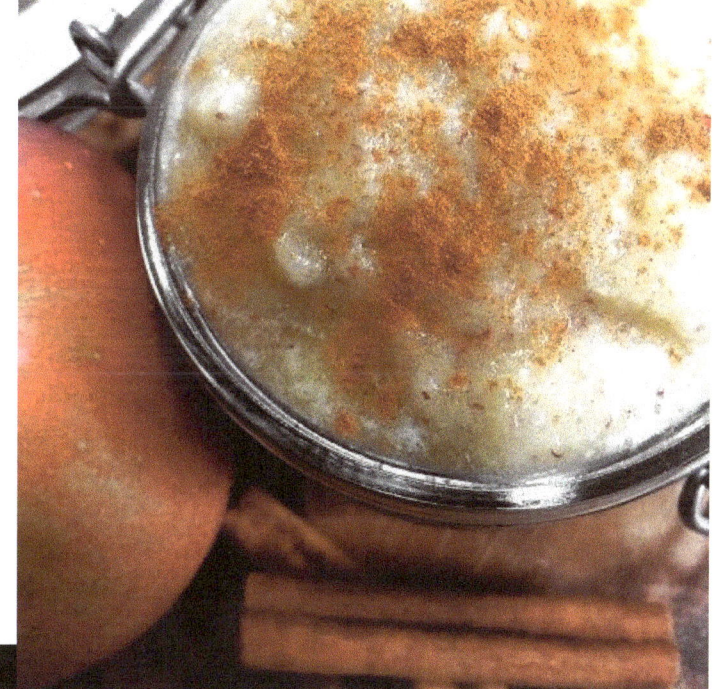

Photo Credit: TableTop Photography, Inc.

DIRECTIONS: place ingredients in blender. Blend until completely smooth.

HANDY TOOLS: blender.

Coco Carob Granola

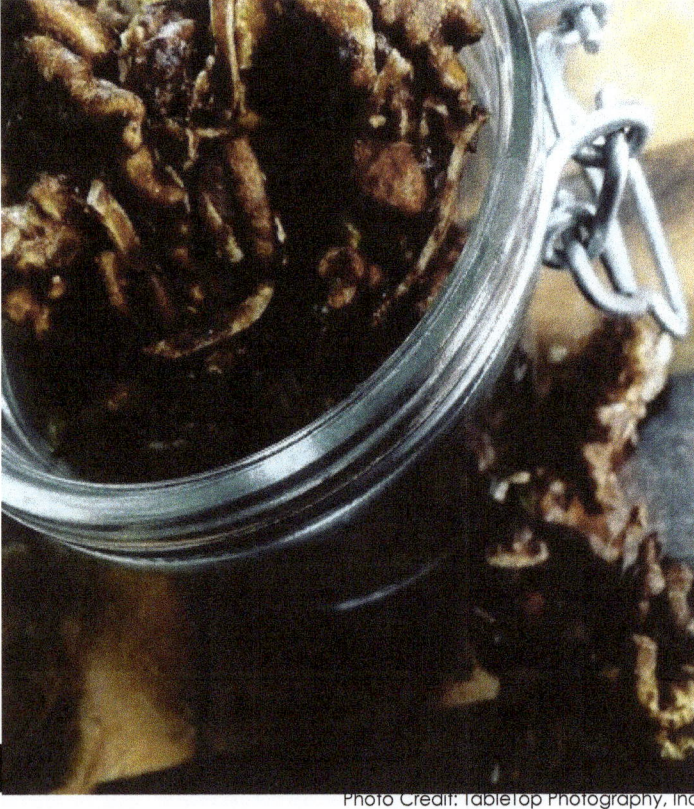

INGREDIENTS:

- 1/2 cup chopped sprouted, dehydrated walnuts (see page 117)
- 1/2 cup chopped sprouted, dehydrated pecans (see page 117)
- 2 Tbsp raw agave or date paste (see page 43)
- 2 Tbsp coconut shreds
- 1 Tbsp raw carob powder (see page 116)
- 1 Tbsp coconut oil
- 1/4 tsp Celtic sea salt

Photo Credit: TableTop Photography, Inc.

DIRECTIONS: place all ingredients together in a medium size bowl and stir until well combined. Place ingredients on a teflex sheet and dehydrate between 95° Fahrenheit (35° Celsius) and 115° Fahrenheit (46° Celsius) for 10 - 12 hours.

HANDY TOOLS: dehydrator and medium size bowl

Coconut Yogurt

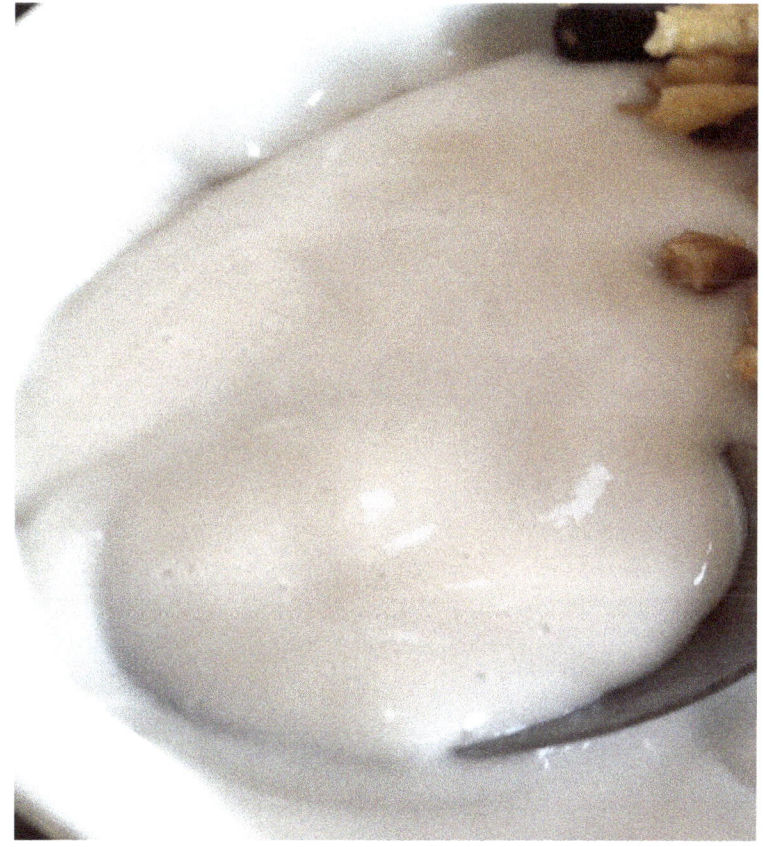

Photo Credit: TableTop Photography, Inc.

INGREDIENTS:

- 1 cup coconut flesh (see page 114)
- 1/4 cup coconut water
- 1 tsp lime juice

DIRECTIONS:
add all ingredients to a blender and blend until smooth. Optional, stir in agave or date paste, granola, and/or fresh fruit to taste.

HANDY TOOLS: blender.

Desserts

Blueberry Cobbler

INGREDIENTS:

- 2 cups fresh blueberries
- 3 Tbsp raw agave or date paste (see page 43)
- 2 Tbsp date sugar
- 1 Tbsp coconut oil
- 1/4 tsp fresh vanilla bean paste (see page 118)
- Crumb Topping (see page 42)

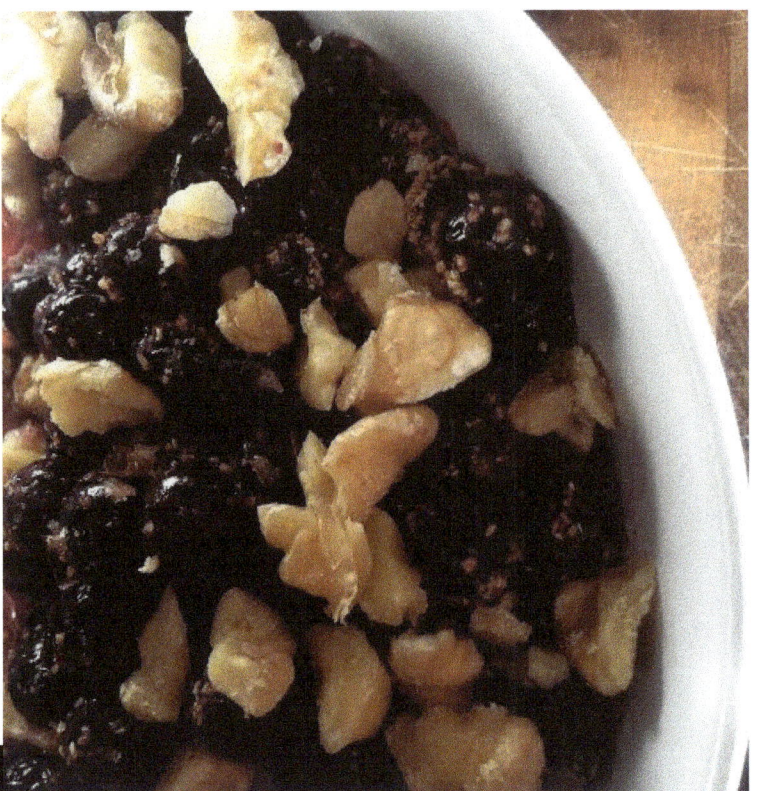

Photo Credit: TableTop Photography, Inc.

DIRECTIONS: place blueberries in a bowl and muddle (smash) them slightly to release their natural juices. Add remaining ingredients (except crumb topping), stir until well combined. Pour contents of bowl into pie dish and top with crumb topping. Dehydrate between 95° Fahrenheit (35° Celsius) and 115° Fahrenheit (46° Celsius) for 2 - 3 hours.

HANDY TOOLS: dehydrator, medium size bowl, and pie dish.

Caramel Apple Crisp

INGREDIENTS:

- 2 apples, medium size
- 1 full batch caramel sauce (see page 35)
- 1 full batch crumb topping (see page 42)

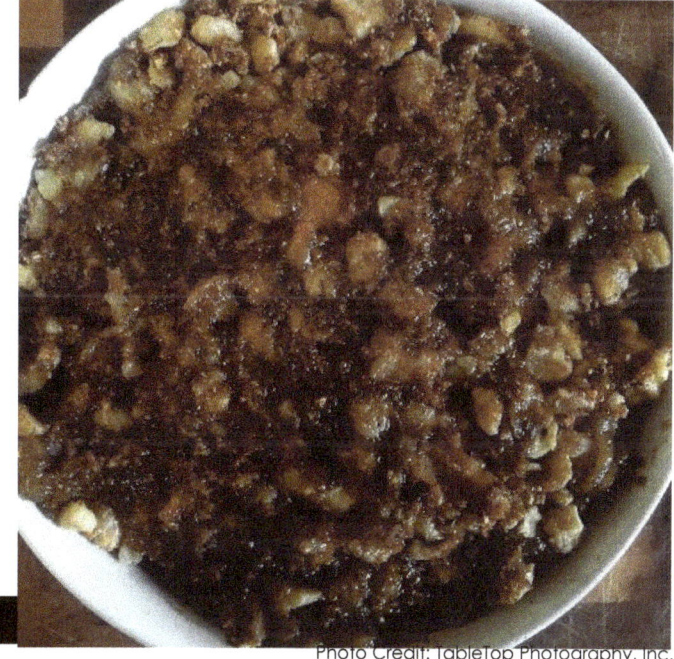

Photo Credit: TableTop Photography, Inc.

DIRECTIONS: place chopped apples in a medium size bowl and pour caramel sauce over apples and stir until well combined. Pour caramel-covered apples in a glass dish and top with crumb topping. Place in dehydrator between 95° Fahrenheit (35° Celsius) and 115° Fahrenheit (46° Celsius) for 2 - 4 hours depending on desired tenderness of apples.

HANDY TOOLS: dehydrator, medium size bowl, and large spoon.

Caramel Pecan Bars

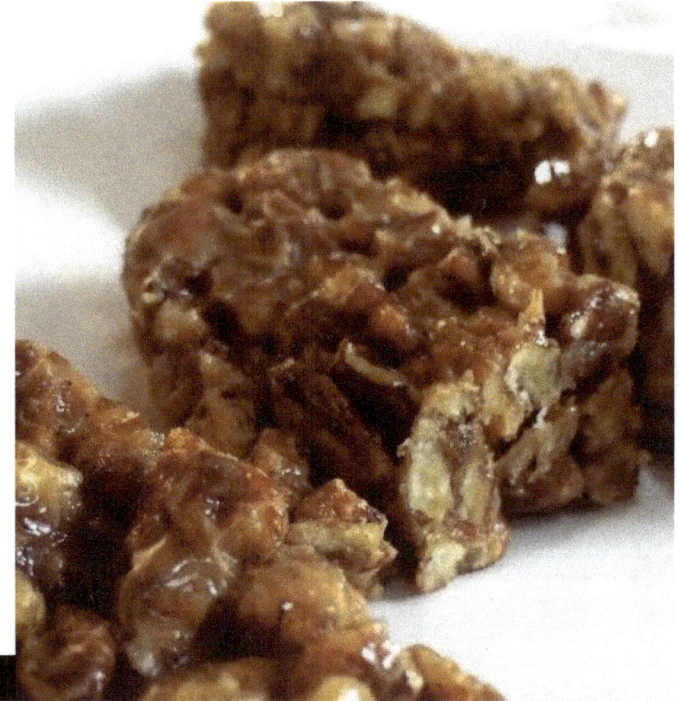

INGREDIENTS:

- 1 cup crushed sprouted, dehydrated pecans (see page 117)
- 1/4 cup caramel sauce (see page 35)
- 1/8 tsp Celtic sea salt or more to taste

DIRECTIONS: stir everything together in a bow then pour into square glass dish. Place in freezer for 4 hours to set. When ready to serve, cut into bars or squares.

HANDY TOOLS: medium size bowl.

Caramel Sauce

INGREDIENTS:

- 1/2 cup chopped dates
- 1/4 cup water
- 1/4 cup coconut oil
- 1/4 cup raw agave or maple syrup (see page 116)
- 2 tsp lucuma powder (see page 115)
- 1 tsp vanilla bean paste (see page 118)
- 1/8 tsp of Celtic sea salt

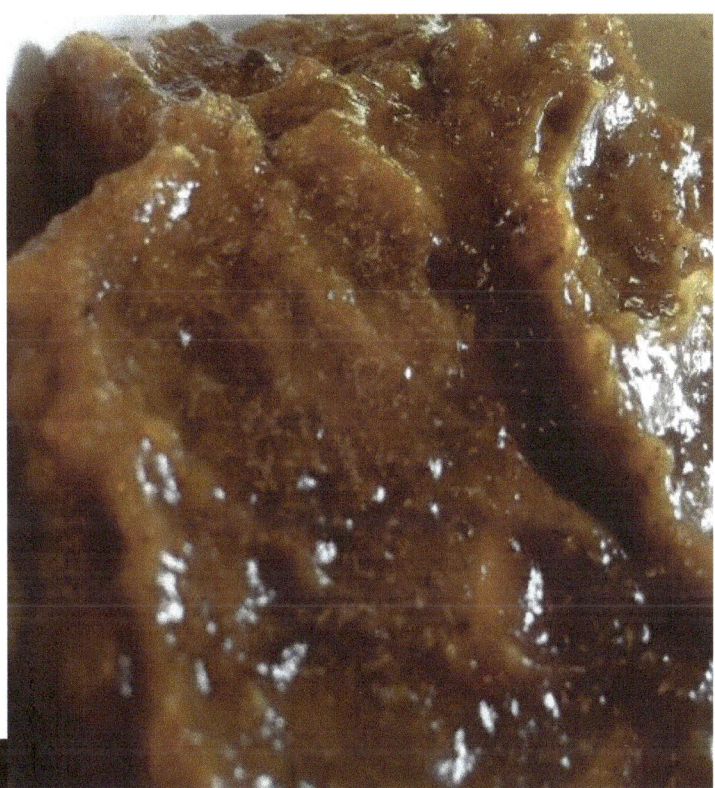

Photo Credit: TableTop Photography, Inc.

DIRECTIONS: place ingredients (except coconut oil) in a food processor and blend until completely smooth, then slowly add coconut oil. Blend until just combined. Store in refrigerator.

HANDY TOOLS: food processor.

Carob Covered Currant Clusters

INGREDIENTS:

- 1/4 cup dried currants
- 1 Tbsp raw carob powder (see page 113)
- 1 Tbsp raw agave or date paste (see page 43)
- 1/4 tsp coconut oil

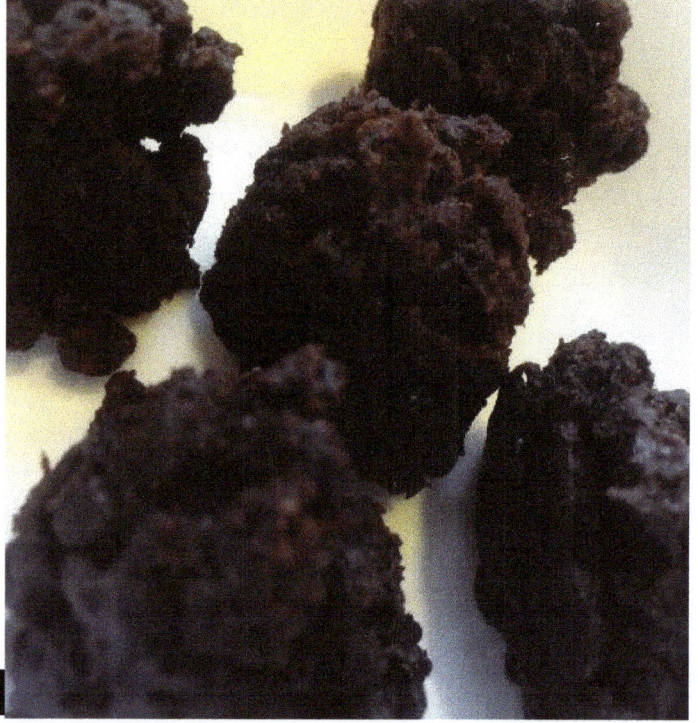

Photo Credit: TableTop Photography, Inc.

DIRECTIONS: place all ingredients in a small bowl and stir until well combined and all of the currants are completely covered.

HANDY TOOLS: small bowl.

Carob Walnut Fudge

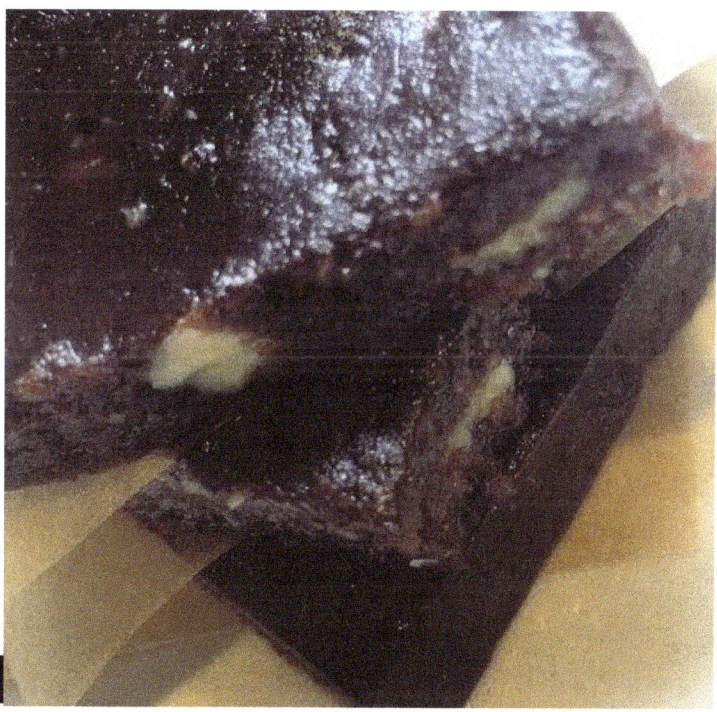

INGREDIENTS:

- 1 cup sprouted, dehydrated walnuts (see page 117)
- 1/2 cup chopped dates
- 2 Tbsp raw carob powder (see page 113)
- 1 Tbsp raw agave or date paste (see page 43)
- 1/8 tsp Celtic sea salt

Photo Credit: TableTop Photography, Inc.

DIRECTIONS: blend all ingredients together in a food processor. While blending, allow fudge batter to form into a ball, then press into a square dish. Chill in refrigerator for 1 hour then cut into squares or as desired.

HANDY TOOLS: food processor.

Cheesecake

INGREDIENTS:

- 1 cup soaked and peeled almonds (see page 117)
- 1/3 cup coconut water or water
- 1/4 cup coconut oil
- 1/4 cup raw agave or date paste (see page 43)
- 1 and 1/2 Tbsp lime juice
- 1/4 tsp fresh vanilla bean paste (see page 118)
- Sweet Pie Crust (see page 50)

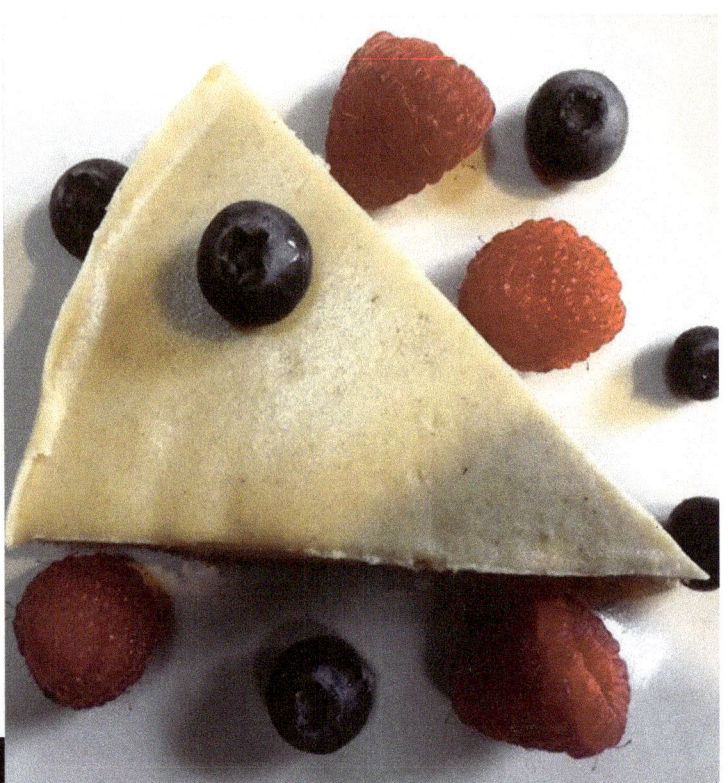

Photo Credit: TableTop Photography, Inc.

DIRECTIONS:
place ingredients in a food processor and blend until completely smooth. Pour into sweet pie crust. Refrigerate for 6 hours or until completely firm.

HANDY TOOLS: food processor.

Coco Banana Crunch Ice Cream

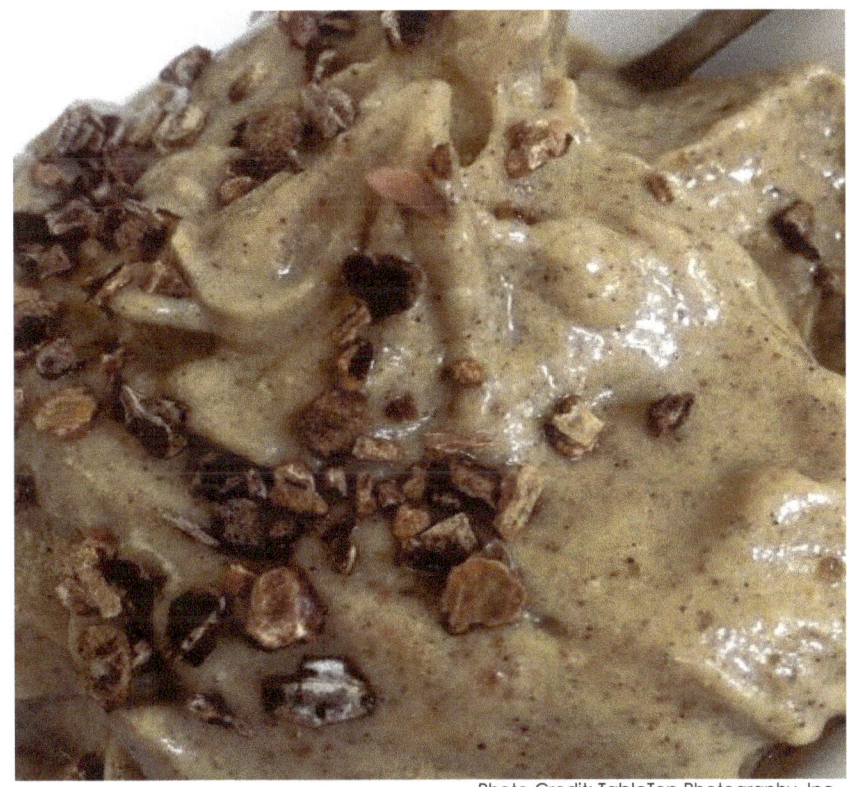

Photo Credit: TableTop Photography, Inc.

INGREDIENTS:

- 1 cup frozen baby bananas
- 1/4 cup packed chopped dates
- 1 Tbsp raw carob powder
- 1 Tbsp raw carob chips

DIRECTIONS:
place all ingredients (except raw carob chips) in food processor. Blend on high until completely smooth. Top with raw carob chips.

HANDY TOOLS:
food processor.

eat! easy everyday raw vegan recipes!

Coconut Bliss Bites

INGREDIENTS:

Coconut Bliss Bites
- 1/2 cup coconut shreds
- 1/4 cup chopped sprouted almonds (see page 117)
- 1/4 cup date paste (see page 43)
- 1/8 tsp Celtic sea salt

Carob Sauce
- 1/4 cup coconut oil
- 2 Tbsp carob powder
- 2 Tbsp raw agave or date paste (see page 43)

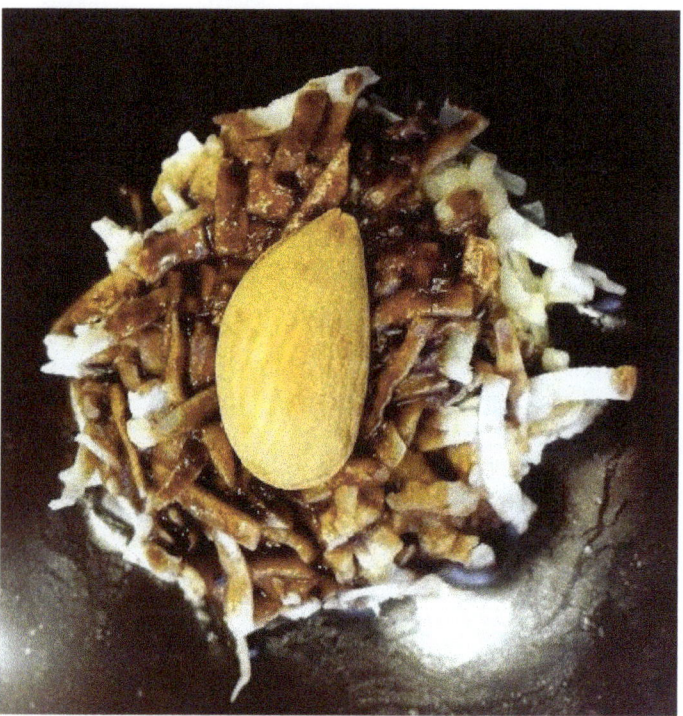

Photo Credit: TableTop Photography, Inc.

DIRECTIONS: place all coconut bliss bites ingredients in a food processor. Blend until smooth then shape into almond drops. Place carob sauce ingredients into a bowl, stir until smooth, and drizzle over the almond bliss bites. Optional, garnish each bliss bite with a dehydrated almond.

HANDY TOOLS: food processor.

Coconut Custard

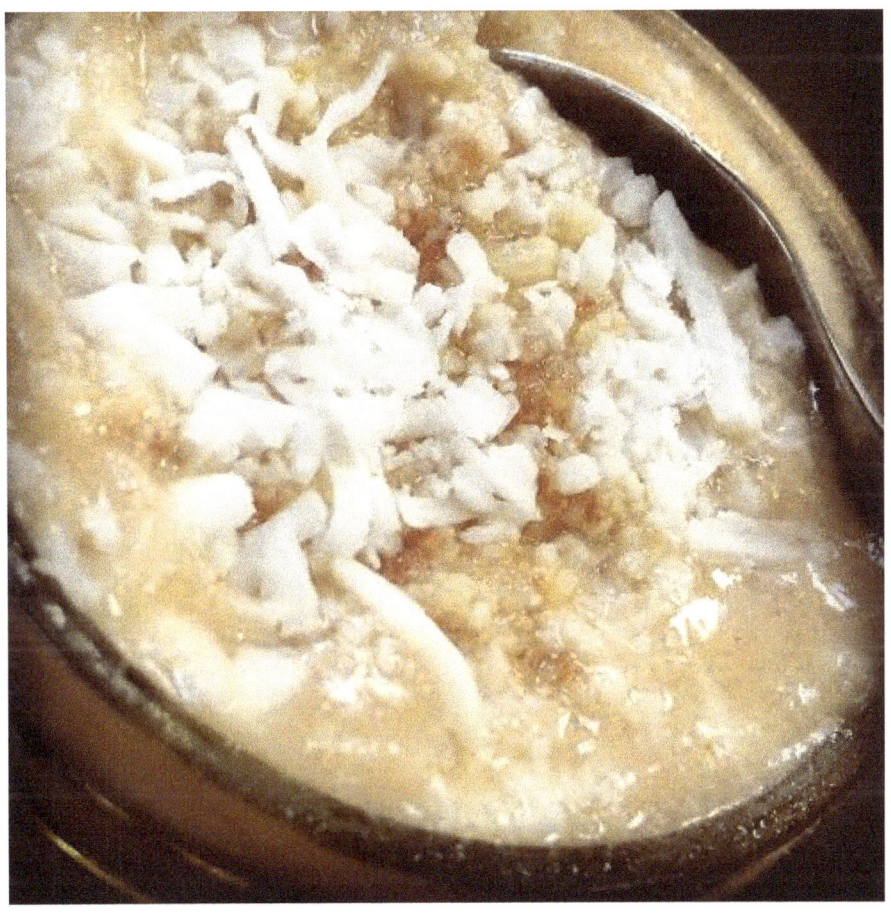

Photo Credit: TableTop Photography, Inc.

INGREDIENTS:

- 1 cup coconut water
- 1 cup coconut flesh (see page 114)
- 1/4 cup chopped dates
- 2 Tbsp coconut oil
- 2 Tbsp coconut shreds

DIRECTIONS:
place all ingredients (except coconut shreds) in a blender and blend until well combined. Garnish with coconut shreds. Place in refrigerator for 2 hours to set.

HANDY TOOLS: blender.

Crumb Topping

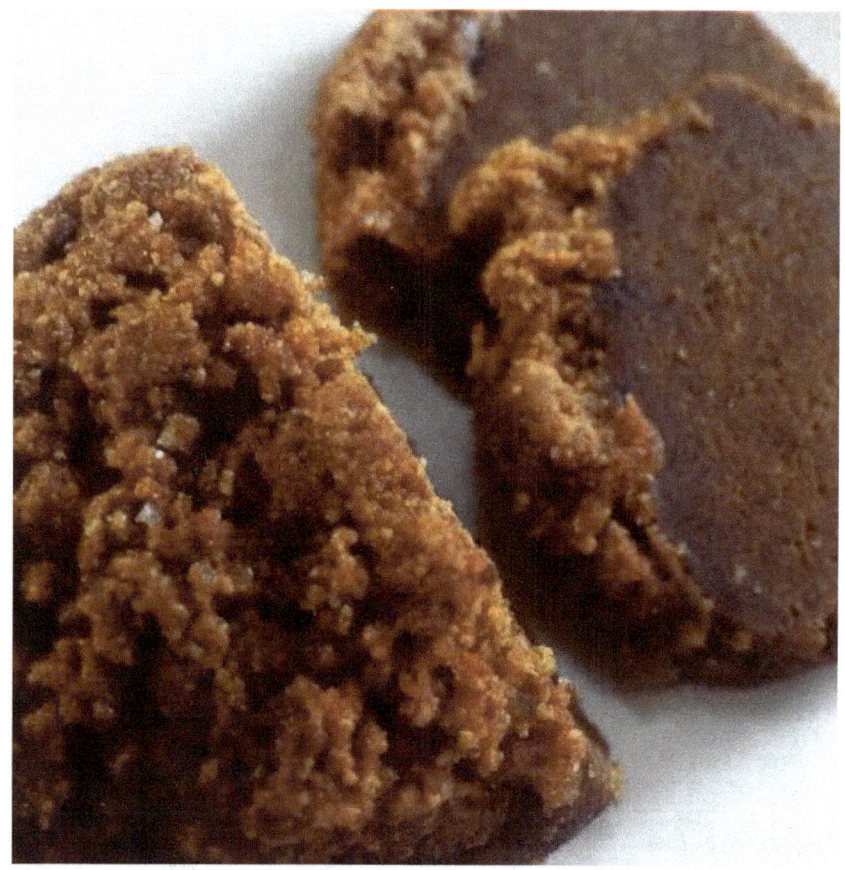

Photo Credit: TableTop Photography, Inc.

INGREDIENTS:

- 1/2 cup sprouted, dehydrated walnuts (see page 117)
- 2 Tbsp raw date sugar (see page 114)
- 1 Tbsp coconut oil
- 1 Tbsp agave or date paste (see page 43)
- 1 tsp cinnamon
- 1/8 tsp of Celtic sea salt

DIRECTIONS:
grind pecans in food processor until fine, then place ground pecans in bowl. Add remaining ingredients to bowl and stir until just combined.

HANDY TOOLS:
food processor and medium size bowl.

eat! easy everyday raw vegan recipes!

Date Paste

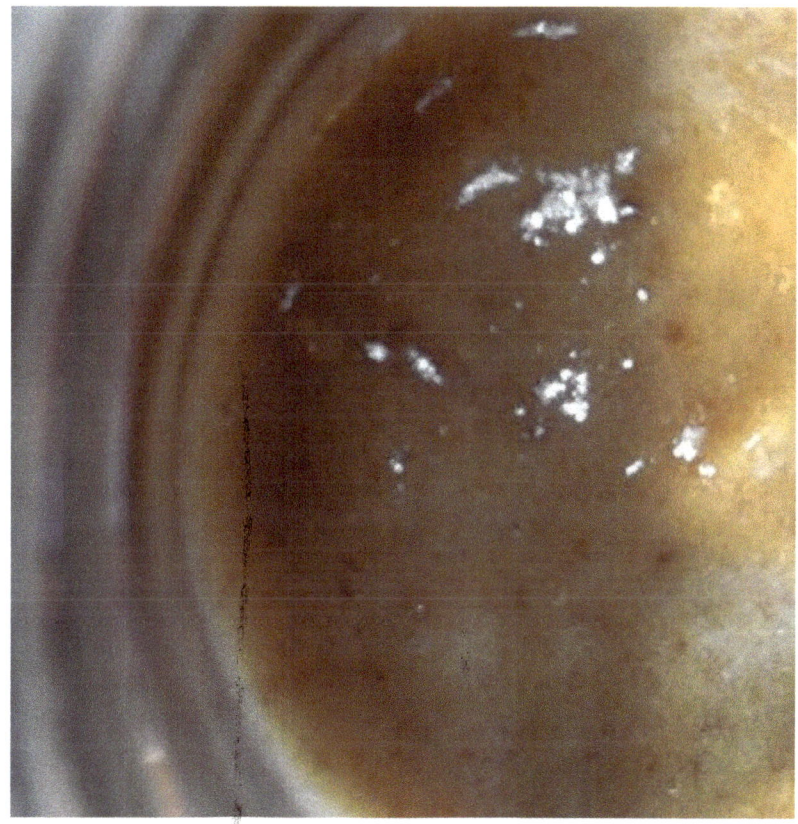

Photo Credit: TableTop Photography, Inc.

INGREDIENTS:

- 1/2 cup chopped dates
- 1/2 cup water

DIRECTIONS:
soak chopped dates in a bowl for 6 hours. After dates have soaked, place dates in blender with 1/4 cup water. Blend until smooth.

HANDY TOOLS:
blender and bowl.

eat! easy everyday raw vegan recipes!

Fresh Berry Sauce

INGREDIENTS:

- 1 cup berries of choice (blackberries, blueberries, etc.)
- 1 Tbsp and 1/2 tsp raw agave or date paste (see page 43)

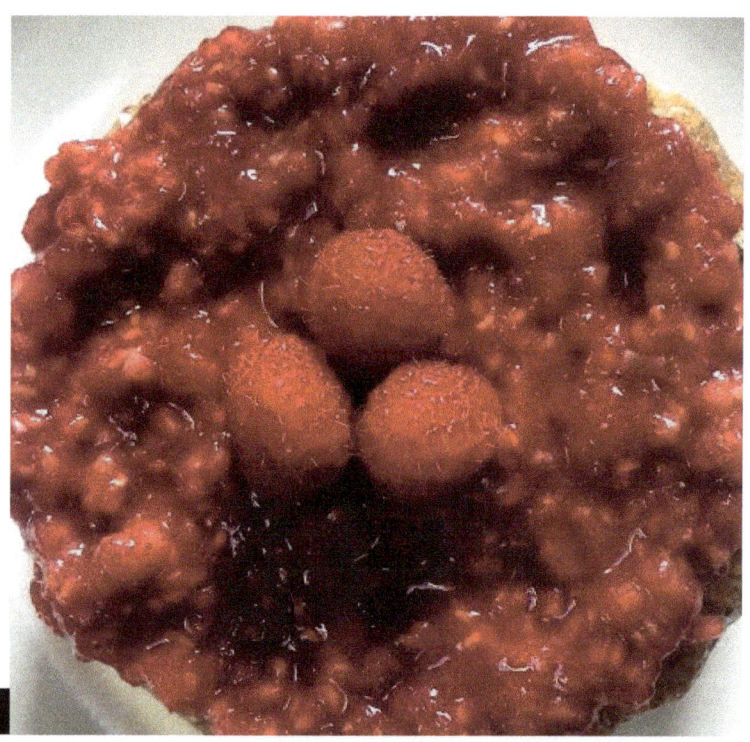

Photo Credit: TableTop Photography, Inc.

DIRECTIONS: place ingredients in a food processor and blend until completely smooth or leave slightly chunky.

HANDY TOOLS: food processor.

Hazelnut Cookie

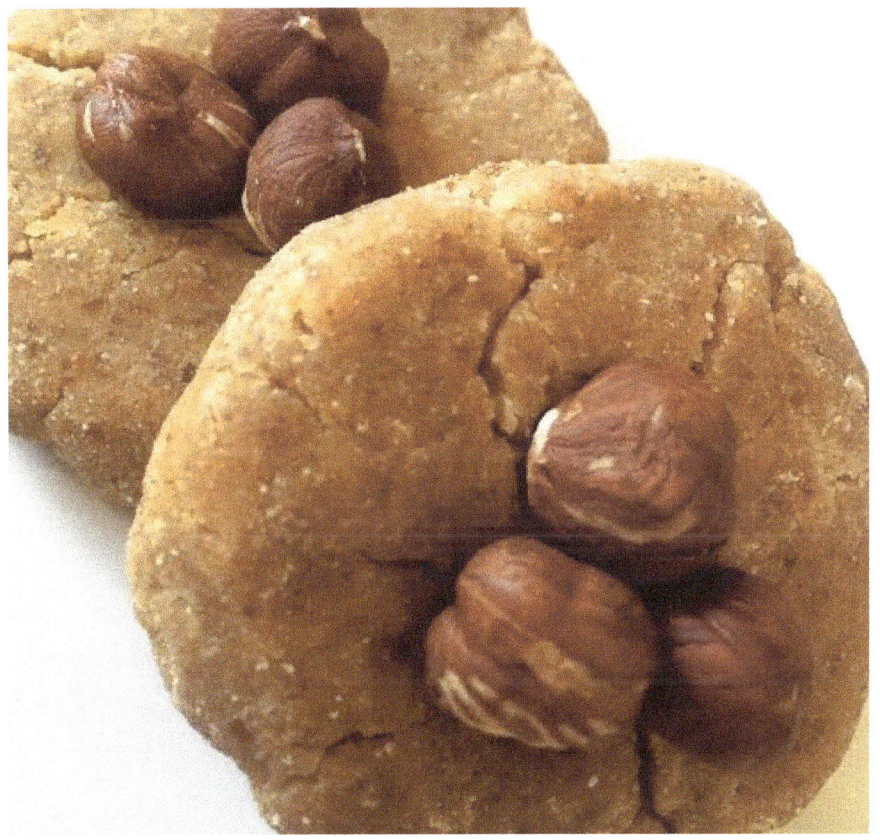

Photo Credit: TableTop Photography, Inc.

INGREDIENTS:

- 1/2 cup dehydrated hazelnut pulp flour (see page 113)
- 1/4 cup chopped dates
- 1/2 tsp cinnamon
- 1/2 tsp fresh vanilla bean paste (see page 118)
- 1/8 tsp Celtic sea salt

DIRECTIONS:
place ingredients in a food processor. Blend until the ingredients form a ball, then shape into cookies.

HANDY TOOLS: food processor.

eat! easy everyday raw vegan recipes!

Key Lime Pie

INGREDIENTS:

- 1 cup coconut flesh (see page 114)
- 1/3 cup lime juice
- 1/2 of a ripe avocado (about 1/3 cup)
- 1/4 cup agave or date paste (see page 43)
- 2 Tbsp coconut oil
- Sweet Pie Crust (see page 50)

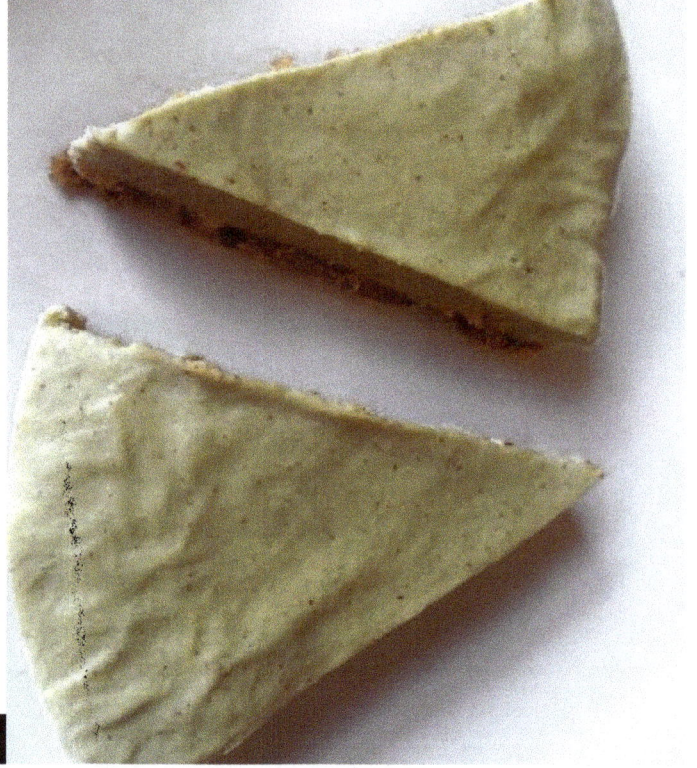

Photo Credit: TableTop Photography, Inc.

DIRECTIONS:
place ingredients in a food processor. Blend until ingredients are well combined, then pour into the sweet pie crust. Place in refrigerator for 6 – 8 hours to set.

HANDY TOOLS: food processor.

Maple Vanilla Frosting

INGREDIENTS:

- 1/4 cup raw agave or date paste (see page 43)
- 1/4 cup coconut butter
- 2 tsp lucuma powder (see page 115)
- 1/2 tsp fresh vanilla bean paste (see page 118)

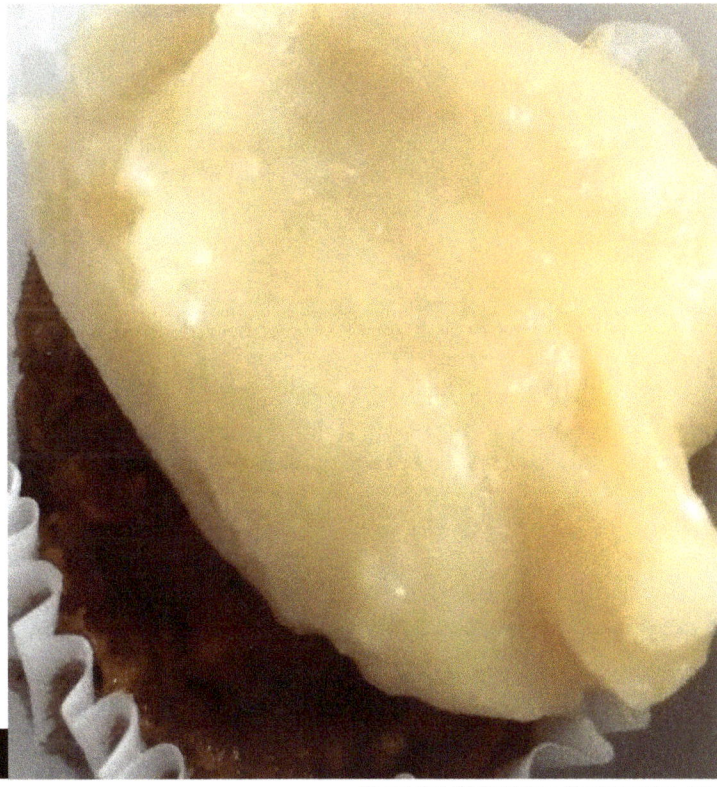

Photo Credit: TableTop Photography, Inc.

DIRECTIONS: place ingredients in a bowl. Blend with a hand-held blender until completely smooth.

HANDY TOOLS: hand-held blender.

Peach Cobbler

INGREDIENTS:

- 2 cups finely chopped ripe peaches
- 2 Tbsp raw agave or date paste (see page 43)
- 2 Tbsp raw date sugar (see page 114)
- 1/8 tsp cinnamon
- Crumb Topping (see page 42)

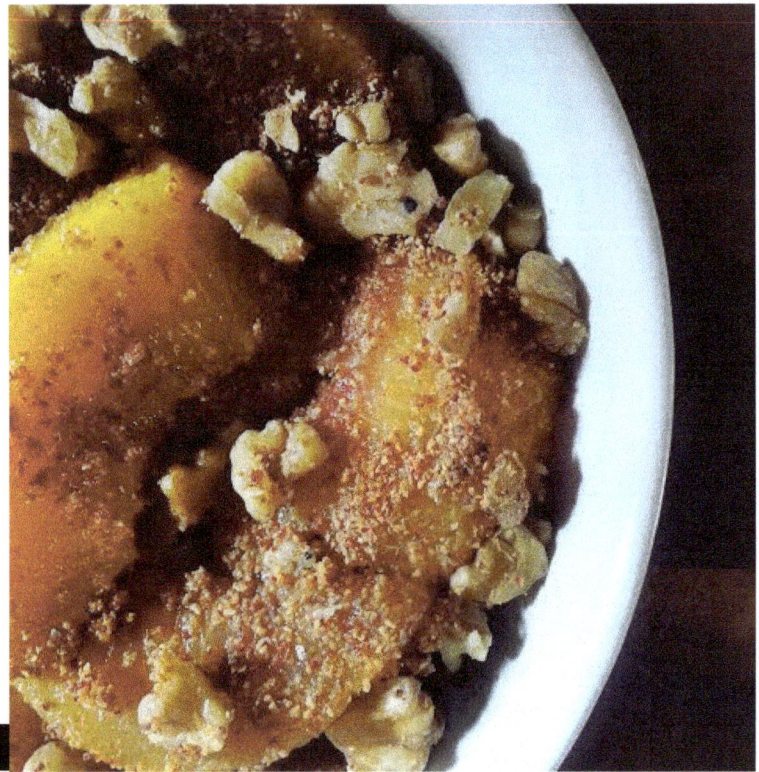

Photo Credit: TableTop Photography, Inc.

DIRECTIONS: place chopped peaches in a bowl and add remaining ingredients (except crumb topping), stir until well combined. Pour contents of bowl into pie dish and top with crumb topping. Dehydrate between 95° Fahrenheit (35° Celsius) and 115° Fahrenheit (46° Celsius) for 1 hour.

HANDY TOOLS: dehydrator, food processor, and medium size bowl.

eat! easy everyday raw vegan recipes!

Pecan Crunch

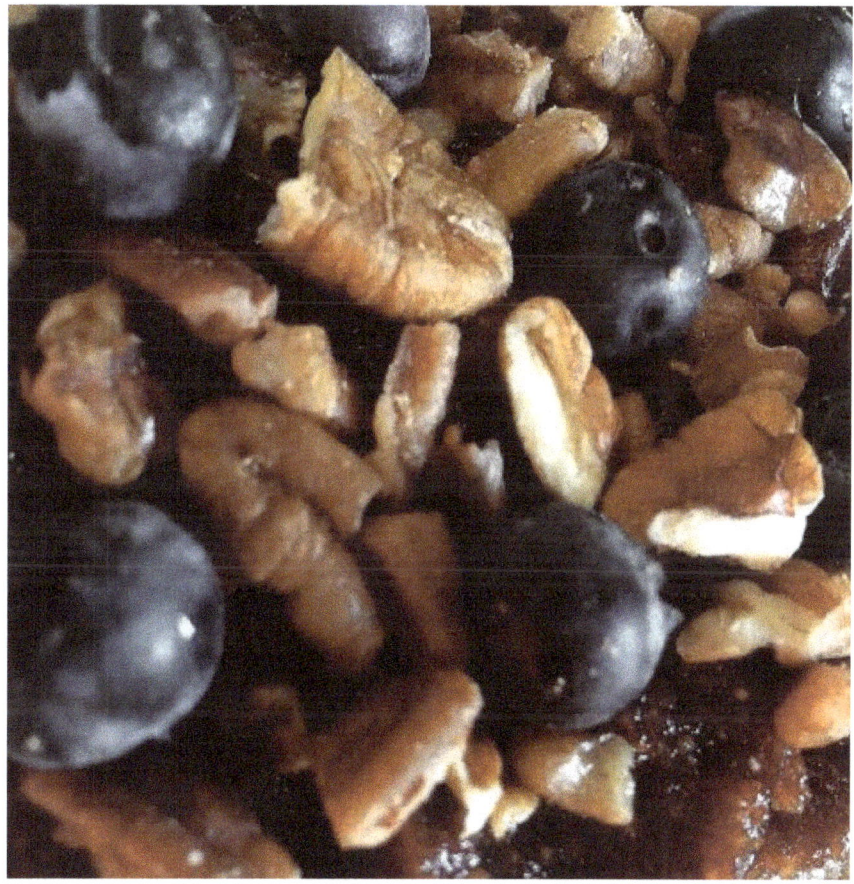

Photo Credit: TableTop Photography, Inc.

INGREDIENTS:

- 1/2 cup sprouted, dehydrated pecans (see page 117)
- 2 Tbsp raw date sugar (see page 114)
- 1 Tbsp raw agave or date paste (see page 43)
- 1/2 tsp cinnamon
- 1/8 tsp Celtic sea salt, or more to taste

DIRECTIONS: place all ingredients together in a food processor and process until a crumble forms.

HANDY TOOLS: food processor.

eat! easy everyday raw vegan recipes!

Sweet Pie Crust

INGREDIENTS:

- 1 cup sprouted, dehydrated walnuts (see page 117)
- 1/2 cup chopped dates
- 1/4 tsp Celtic sea salt

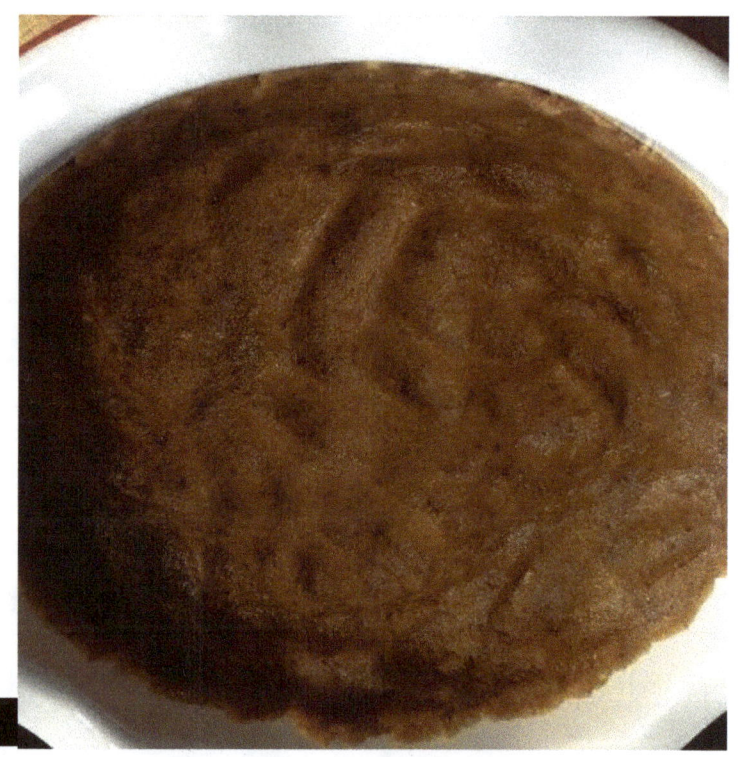

Photo Credit: TableTop Photography, Inc.

DIRECTIONS: place ingredients in a food processor. Blend until the ingredients form a ball, then press the ball into a pie dish. Use for your favorite sweet pie filling.

HANDY TOOLS: food processor and pie dish.

Vanilla Bean Pudding

INGREDIENTS:

- 3/4 cup coconut flesh (see page 114)
- 1/2 cup water
- 1/4 cup chopped dates
- 1/4 tsp fresh vanilla bean paste (see page 118)

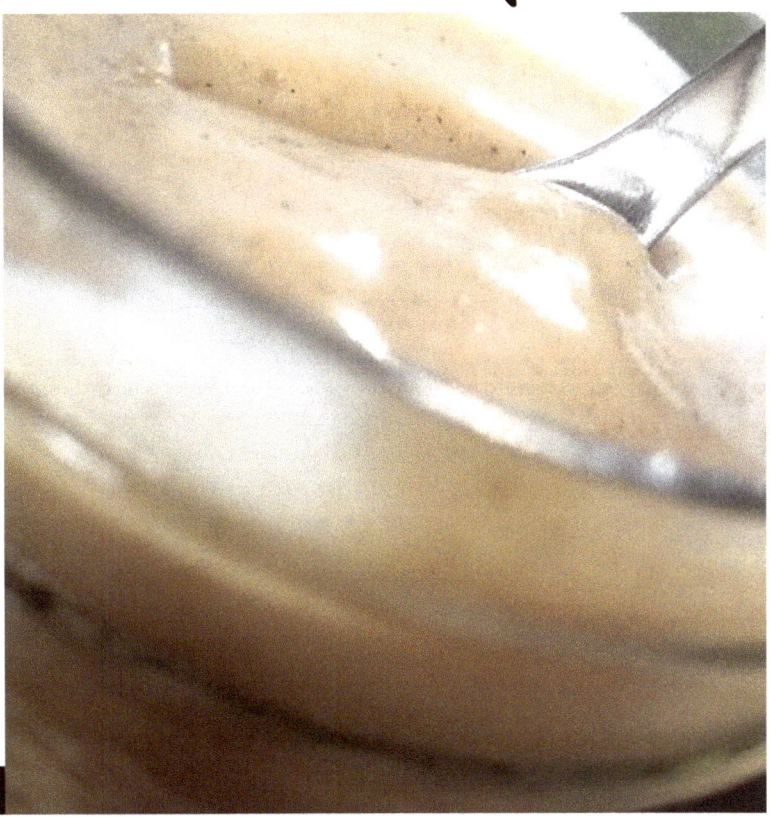

Photo Credit: TableTop Photography, Inc.

DIRECTIONS:
place all ingredients in a blender and blend until well combined. Place in refrigerator for 2 hours to set.

HANDY TOOLS: blender.

Dips, Sauces, & Spreads

Alfredo Sauce

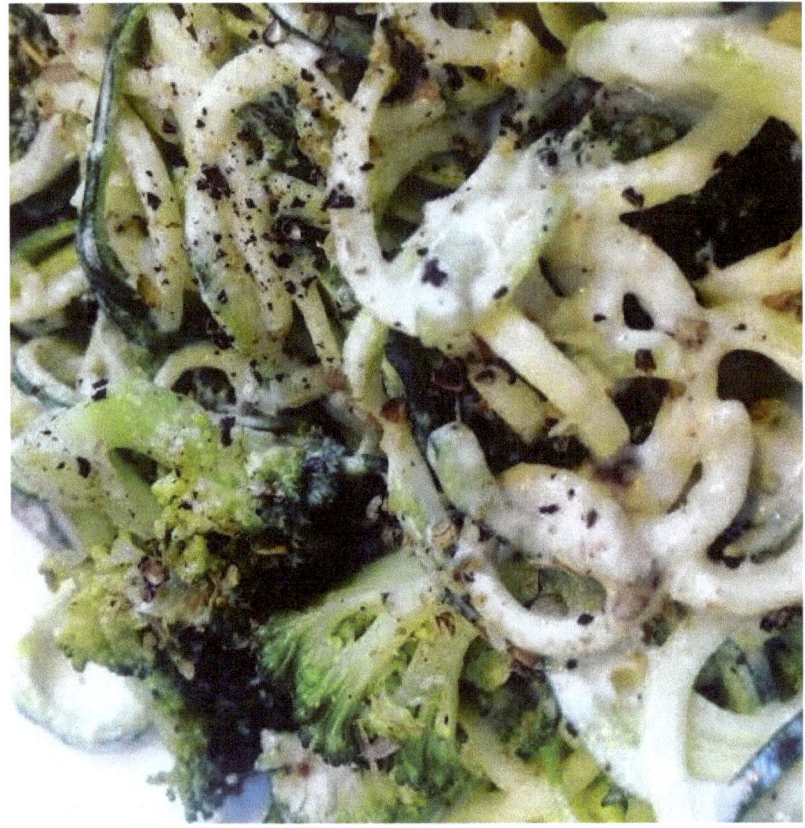

Photo Credit: TableTop Photography, Inc.

INGREDIENTS:

- 1 cup macadamia nuts
- 1 cup water
- 1/2 Tbsp apple cider vinegar
- 1/2 Tbsp raw agave or date paste (see page 43)
- 2 tsp onion powder
- 1/2 tsp Celtic sea salt

DIRECTIONS: blend ingredients until smooth and creamy.

HANDY TOOLS: blender.

Buttery Pasta Sauce

INGREDIENTS:

- 4 Tbsp olive oil
- 5 grated macadamia nuts
- 1/2 tsp sage
- 1/2 tsp thyme
- 1/2 tsp oregano
- 1/2 tsp basil
- 1/4 tsp Celtic sea salt

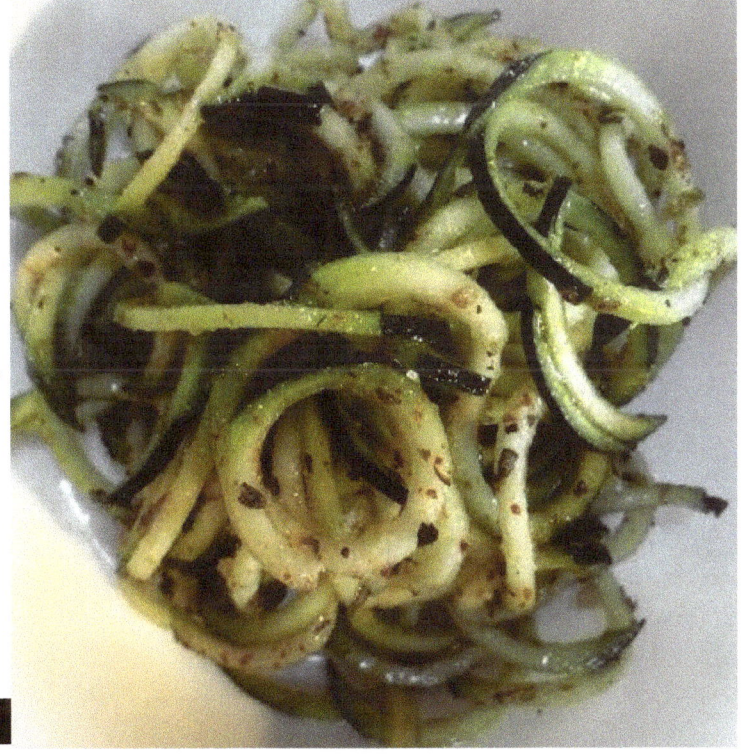

Photo Credit: TableTop Photography, Inc.

DIRECTIONS: add all ingredients to a bowl and whisk together.

HANDY TOOLS: small bowl and whisk.

eat! easy everyday raw vegan recipes!

Coconut Curry Sauce

INGREDIENTS:

- 2 Tbsp coconut oil
- 1 Tbsp curry powder
- 2 tsp onion powder
- 1/4 tsp Celtic sea salt

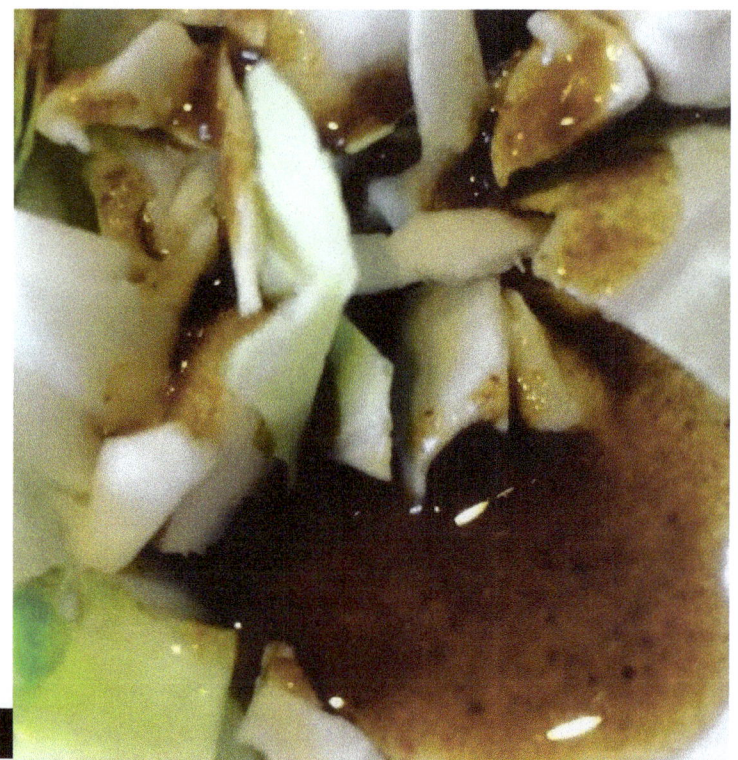

Photo Credit: TableTop Photography, Inc.

DIRECTIONS: place all ingredients in a bowl and whisk together to combine.

HANDY TOOLS: small bowl and whisk.

Concord Grape Jelly

INGREDIENTS:

- 1/2 cup Concord grapes
- 1/4 cup chopped dates
- 1 tsp psyllium husk (see page 117)

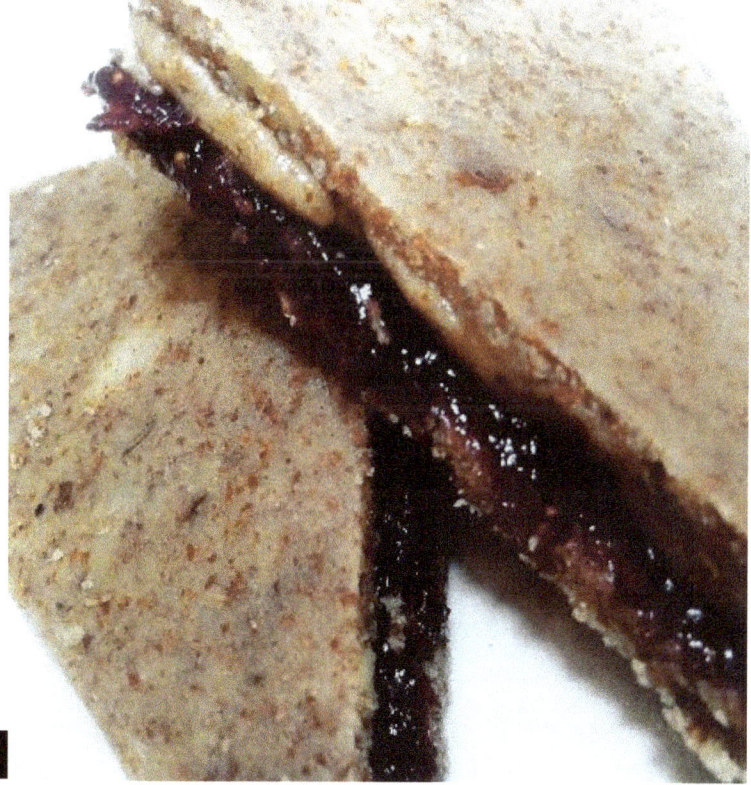
Photo Credit: TableTop Photography, Inc.

DIRECTIONS: place ingredients in blender. Blend until completely smooth.

HANDY TOOLS: blender.

eat! easy everyday raw vegan recipes!

Creamy Dill

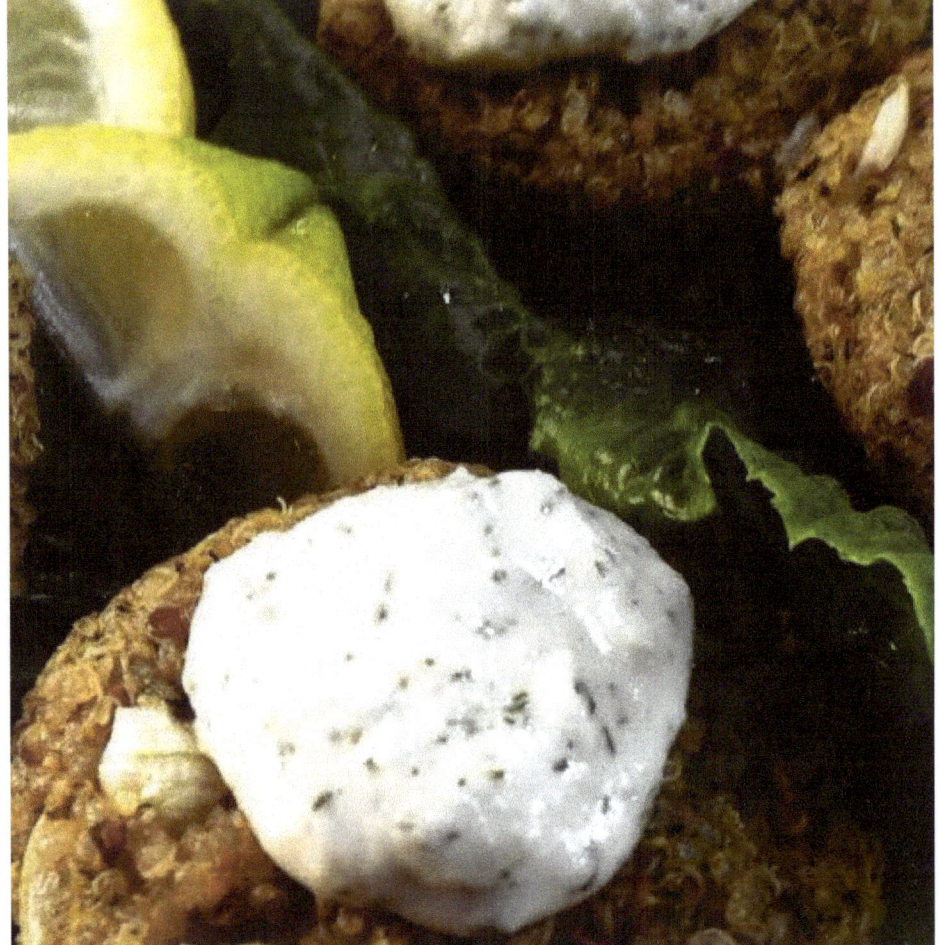

Photo Credit: TableTop Photography, Inc.

INGREDIENTS:

- 1/2 cup soaked and peeled almonds (see page 117)
- 1/3 cup water
- 1 tsp dried dill
- 1/4 tsp Celtic sea salt

DIRECTIONS: blend all ingredients in a blender until completely smooth.

HANDY TOOLS: blender.

Easy Vinaigrette

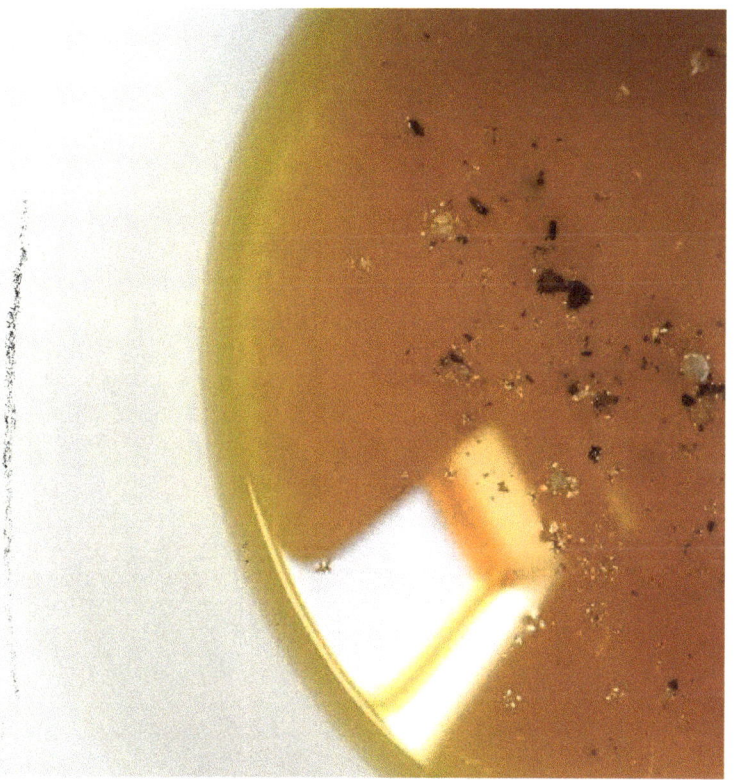

Photo Credit: TableTop Photography, Inc.

INGREDIENTS:

- 1/4 cup apple cider vinegar
- 1/4 cup olive oil
- 2 Tbsp water
- 2 Tbsp raw agave or date paste (see page 43)
- 1/4 tsp onion powder
- 1/4 tsp crushed red pepper flakes (optional)
- 1/8 tsp Celtic sea salt

DIRECTIONS: place all ingredients together in a small bowl and whisk vigorously until well combined.

HANDY TOOLS: small bowl and whisk.

eat! easy everyday raw vegan recipes!

Honey Butter

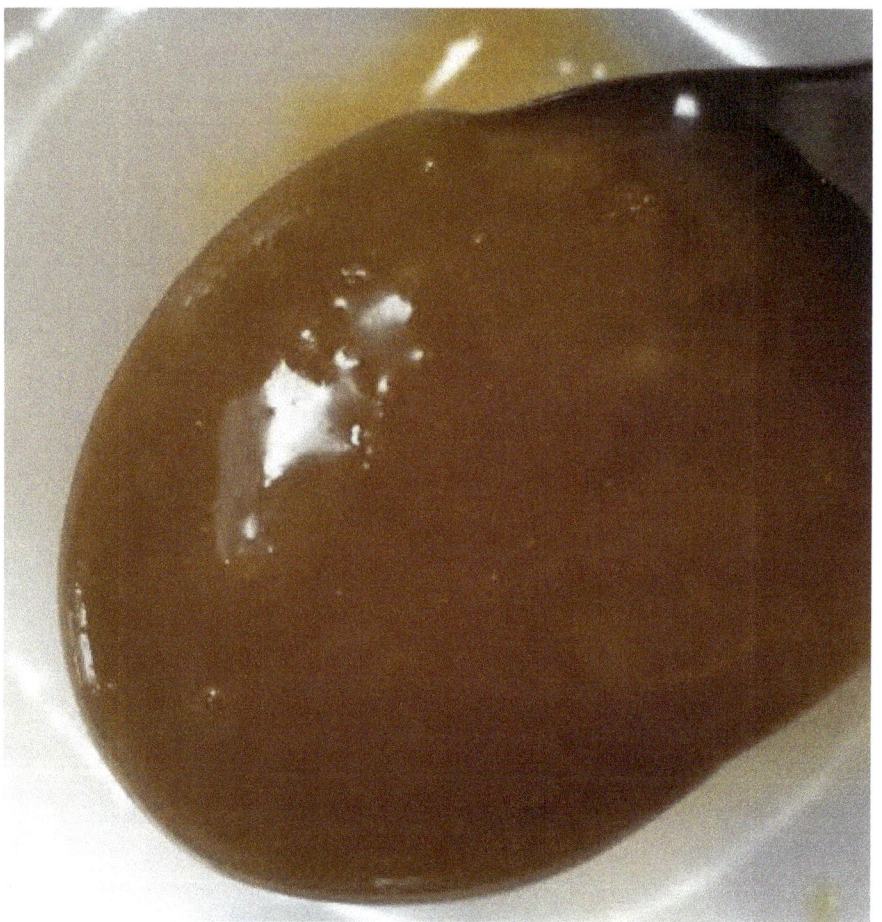

Photo Credit: TableTop Photography, Inc.

INGREDIENTS:

- 1 Tbsp coconut oil
- 1 tsp raw honey (*see page 115)
- Pinch of Celtic sea salt

DIRECTIONS:
stir in a small bowl until well combined and place in fridge for 30 minutes to firm up.

HANDY TOOLS: small bowl.

Italian Dressing

INGREDIENTS:

- 1/4 cup olive oil
- 2 Tbsp apple cider vinegar
- 1 Tbsp raw agave or date paste (see page 43)
- 1/2 Tbsp oregano
- 1/2 tsp basil
- 1/4 tsp sage
- 1/4 tsp thyme
- 1/4 tsp onion powder
- 1/4 tsp Celtic sea salt

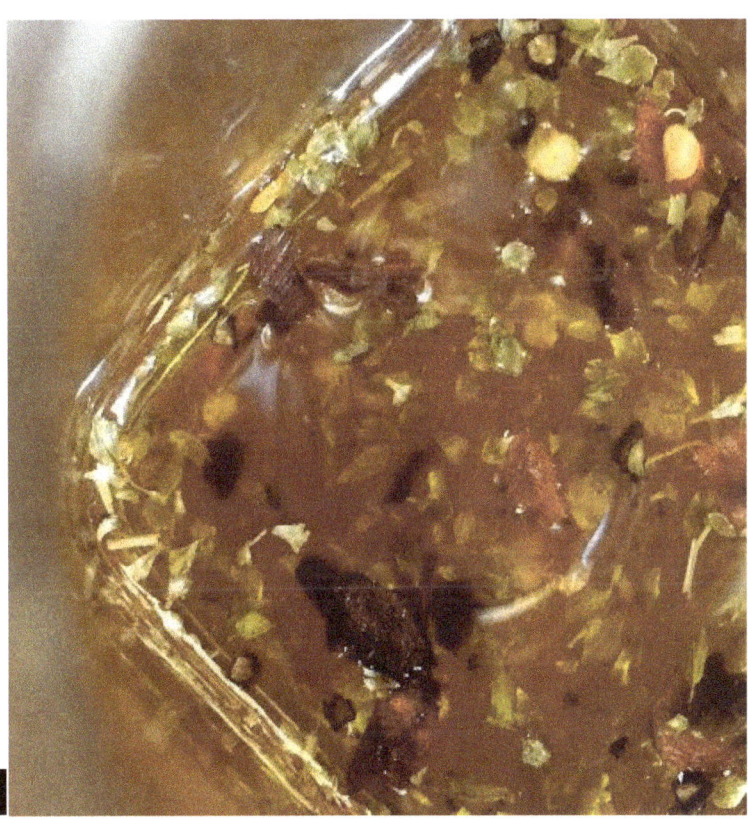

Photo Credit: TableTop Photography, Inc.

DIRECTIONS: add all ingredients to a bowl and whisk vigorously.

HANDY TOOLS: small bowl and whisk.

Peach Preserves

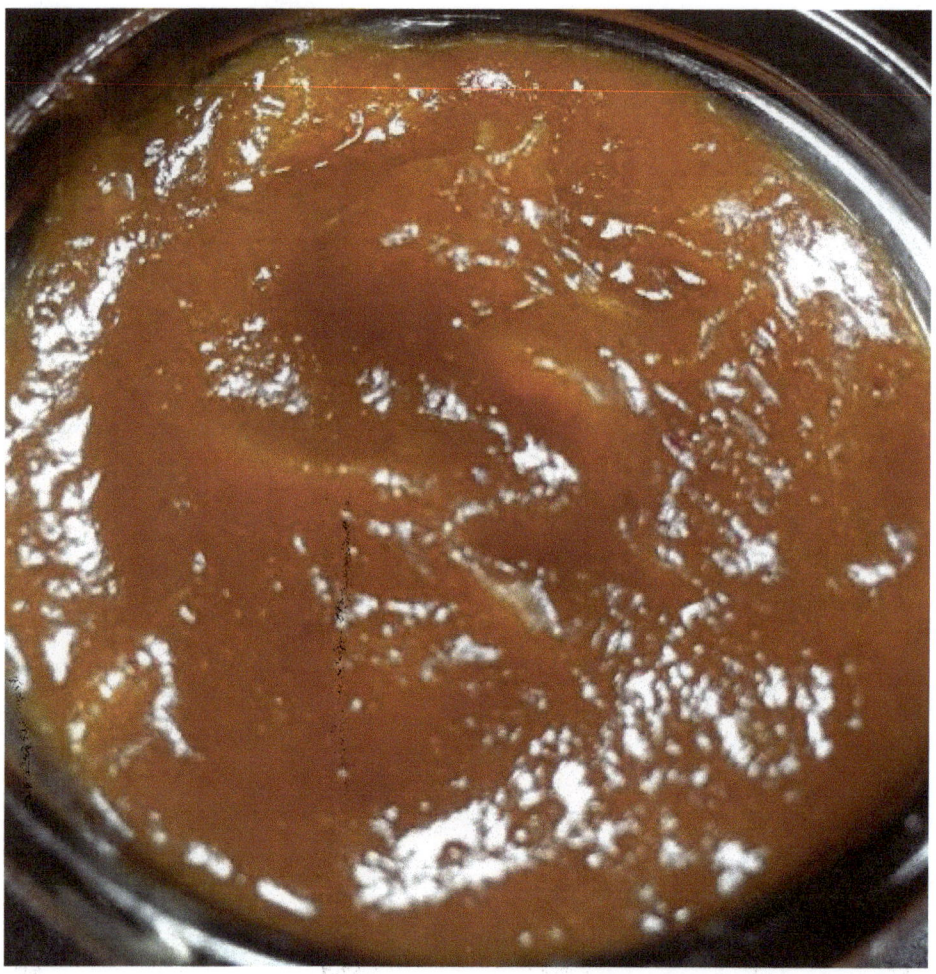

Photo Credit: TableTop Photography, Inc.

INGREDIENTS:

- 1 cup chopped ripe yellow peaches
- 2 Tbsp chopped dates
- 1 tsp psyllium husk (see page 117)
- 1/4 tsp lime juice

DIRECTIONS:
place all ingredients in a blender and blend until well combined. Place in refrigerator for 2 hours to set.

HANDY TOOLS: blender.

Sage & Mushroom Gravy

INGREDIENTS:

- 2 cups chopped mushroom
- 1/2 cup water
- 2 Tbsp olive oil
- 1 Tbsp sage
- 2 tsp onion powder
- 1 tsp Celtic sea salt
- 1 tsp thyme

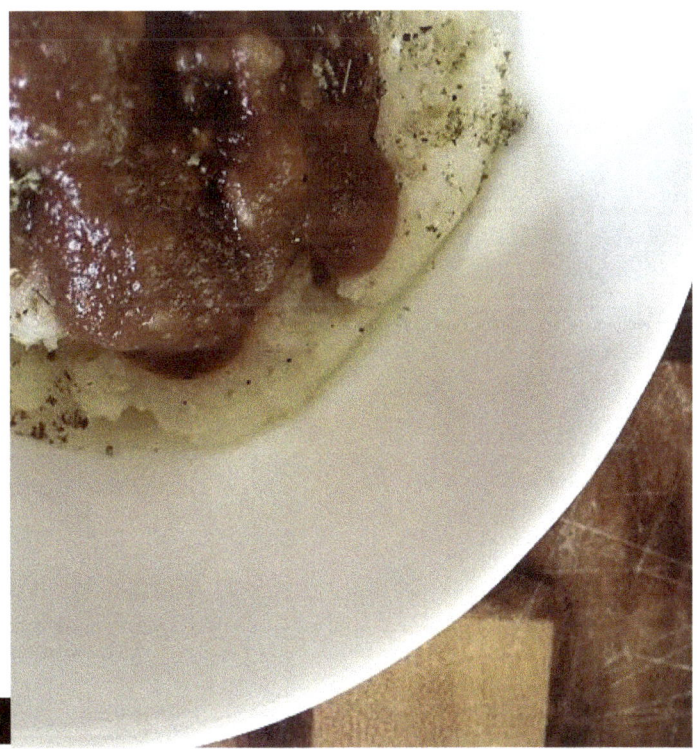

Photo Credit: TableTop Photography, Inc.

DIRECTIONS: place all ingredients (except thyme) in a blender and blend until smooth and creamy. Gently stir in thyme.

HANDY TOOLS: blender.

Sesame Seed & Scallion Hummus

INGREDIENTS:

- 2 cups soaked & sprouted chickpeas (see page 119)
- 1/3 cup tahini butter (see page 66)
- 1/4 cup olive oil
- 1 Tbsp onion powder
- 1 tsp Celtic sea salt

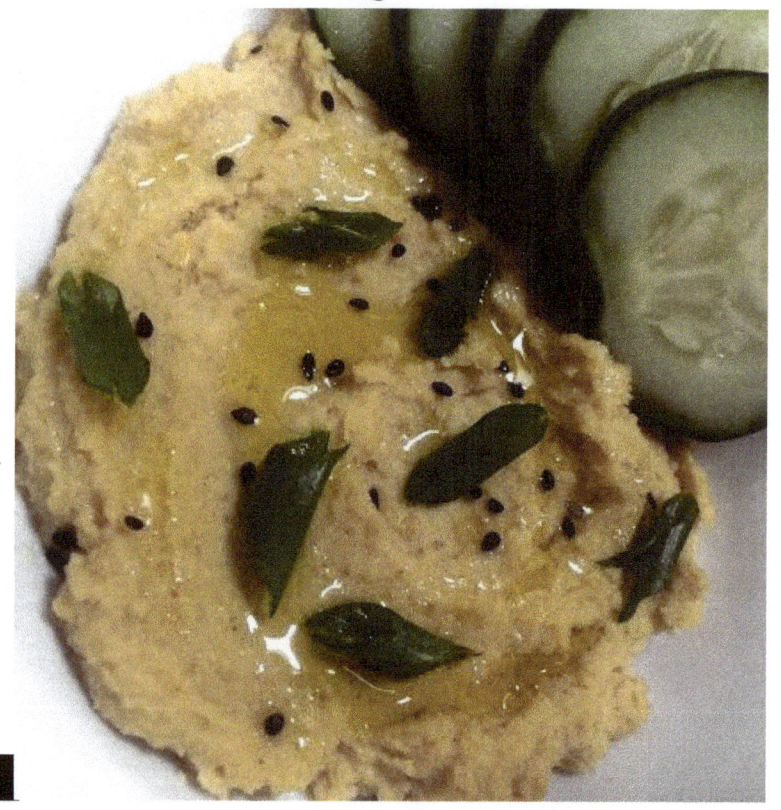

Photo Credit: TableTop Photography, Inc.

DIRECTIONS: place all ingredients in food processor and blend until completely smooth. To serve, garnish with fresh sliced scallions, black sesame seeds (optional), and a drizzle of olive oil.

HANDY TOOLS: food processor.

Spicy Salsa

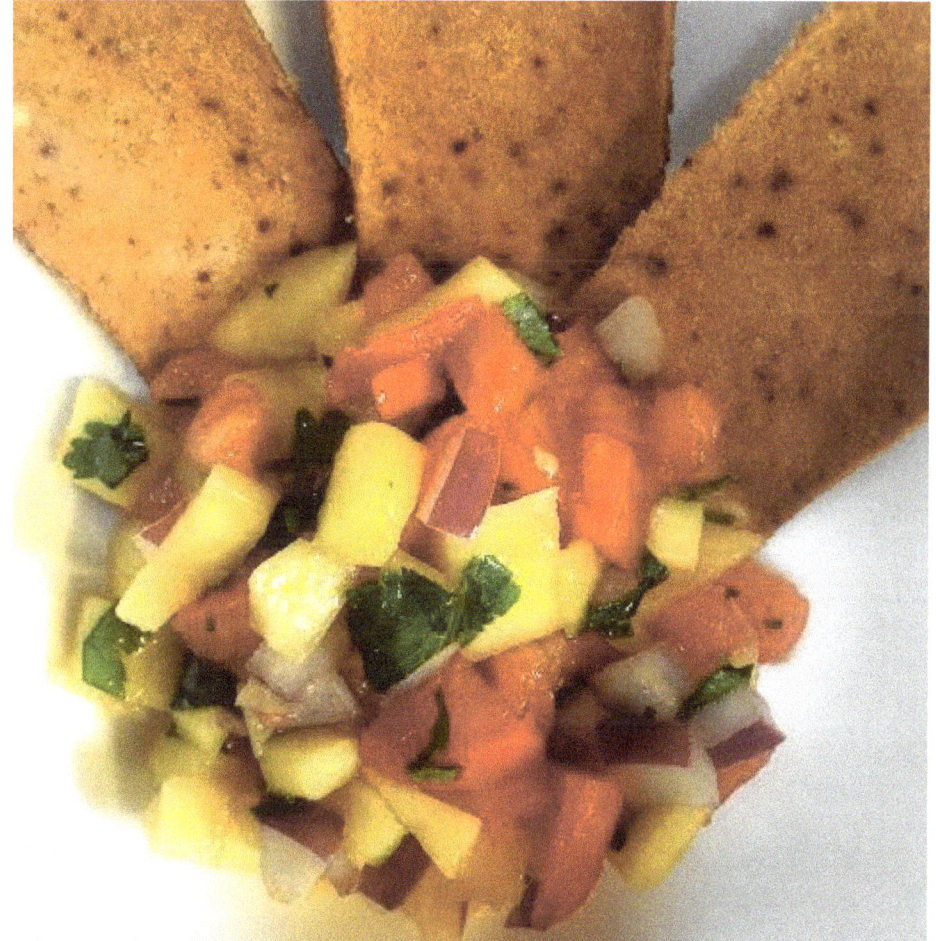

Photo Credit: TableTop Photography, Inc.

INGREDIENTS:

- 1 cup cherry tomatoes
- 1/4 cup chopped cilantro
- 2 Tbsp chopped red onion
- 2 tsp fresh lime juice
- 1/2 tsp Celtic sea salt
- 1/4 tsp crushed red pepper flakes

DIRECTIONS:
stir all ingredients together in a bowl and let sit in fridge to chill. Optional, add chopped mango.

HANDY TOOLS:
food processor.

eat! easy everyday raw vegan recipes!

Tahini Butter

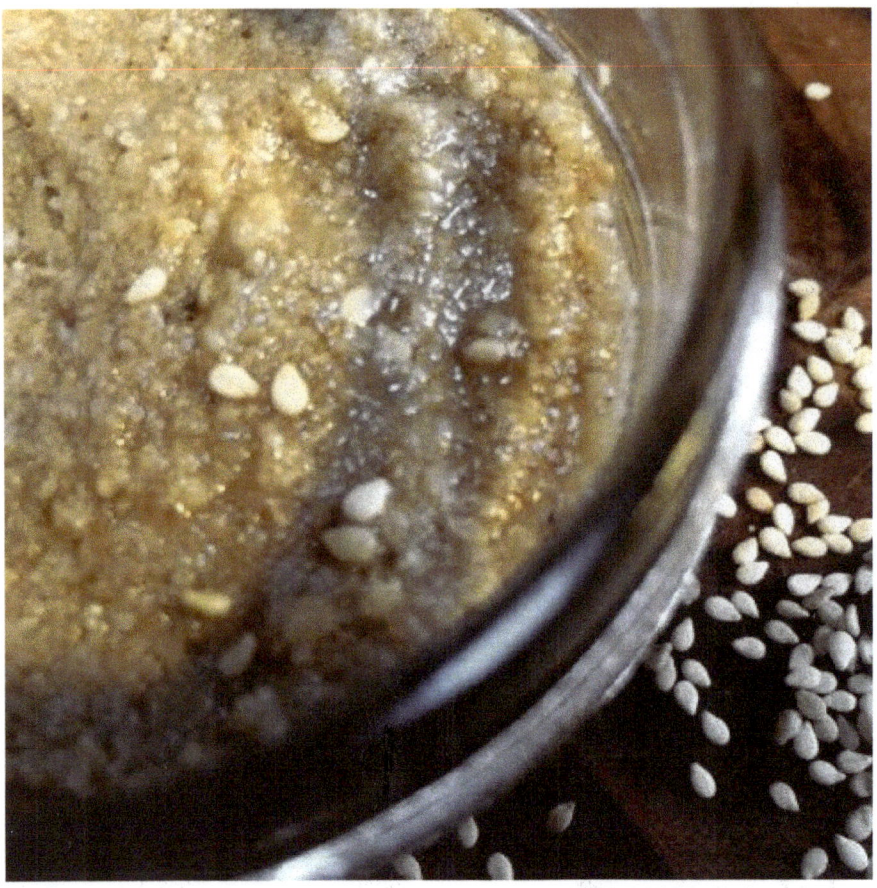

Photo Credit: TableTop Photography, Inc.

INGREDIENTS:

- 1 cup brown or white sesame seeds
- 1/4 cup sesame oil
- 1/4 tsp Celtic sea salt

DIRECTIONS: add all ingredients to a food processor and blend until completely smooth.

HANDY TOOLS: food processor.

Tahini Dressing

INGREDIENTS:

- 1 cup water
- 1/3 cup tahini butter (see page 66)
- 2 tsp onion powder
- 1 tsp lime juice
- 1/2 tsp Celtic sea salt

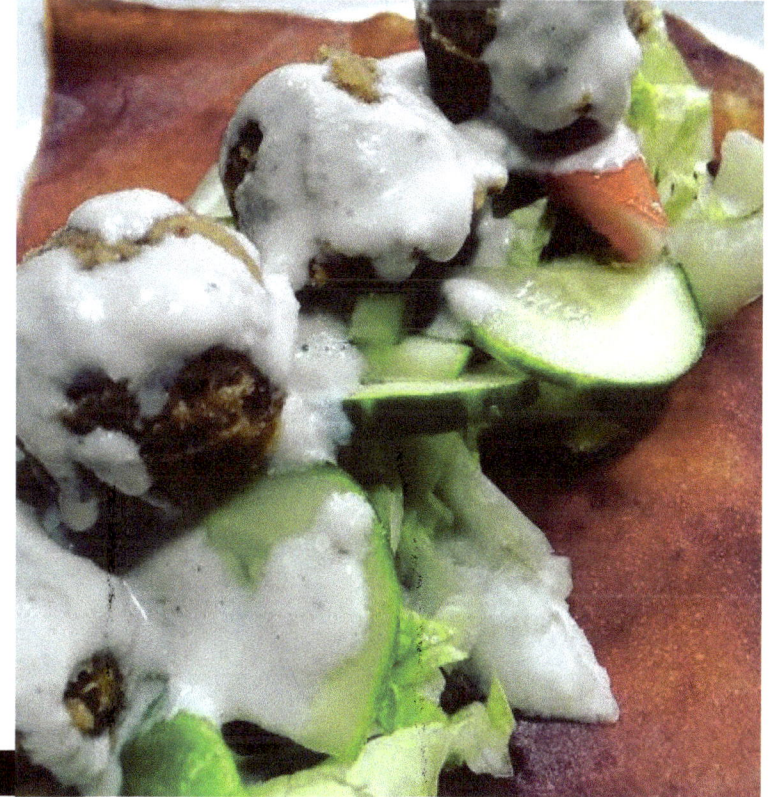

Photo Credit: TableTop Photography, Inc.

DIRECTIONS: place all ingredients in a blender and blend until completely smooth.

HANDY TOOLS: blender.

Tomato Basil Sauce

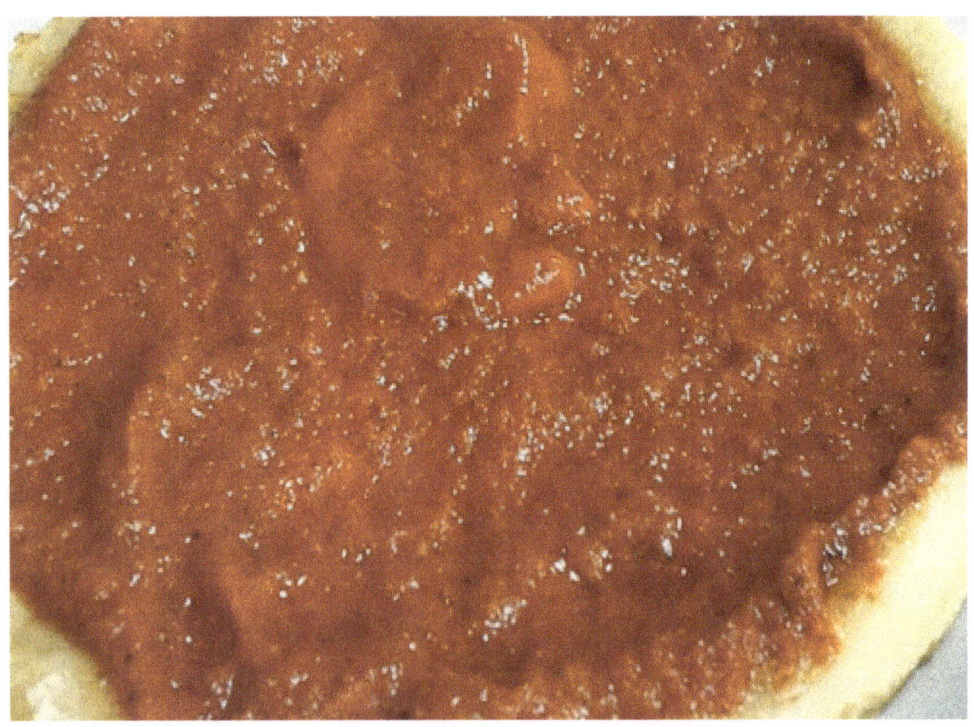

Photo Credit: TableTop Photography, Inc.

INGREDIENTS:

- 1 cup chopped cherry or Roma tomatoes
- 2 Tbsp dried basil
- 2 Tbsp olive oil
- 1/2 tsp Celtic sea salt

DIRECTIONS: place all of the ingredients together in a blender and blend until completely smooth.

HANDY TOOLS: blender.

Entrées

BBQ Vegetable Medley

INGREDIENTS:

- 4 cups of assorted chopped vegetables (zucchini, summer squash, broccoli, peppers, cabbage)
- 1/3 cup water
- 3 Tbsp olive oil
- 1 Tbsp BBQ seasoning
- 1 Tbsp onion powder
- 1/4 tsp Celtic sea salt

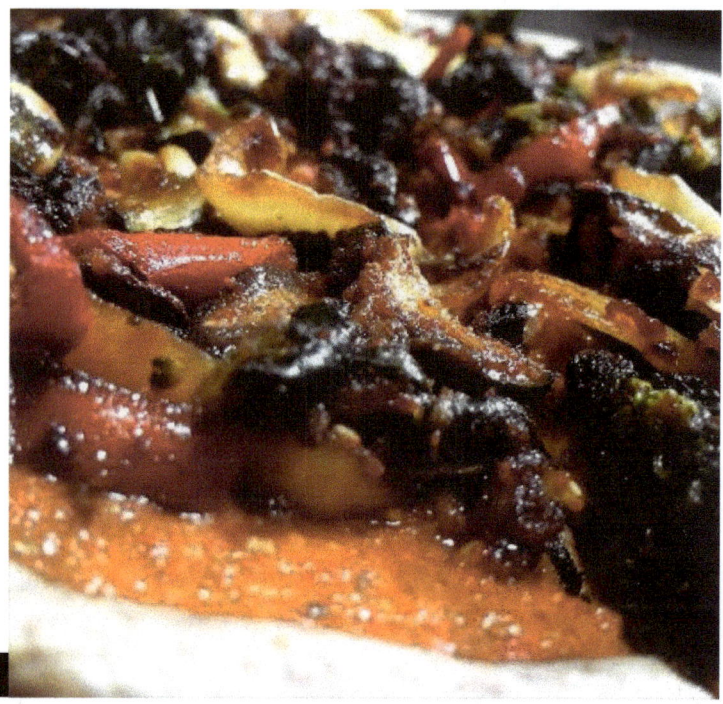

Photo Credit: TableTop Photography, Inc.

DIRECTIONS: place all ingredients together in a large shallow glass (or ceramic) dish and stir until well combined. Dehydrate between 95° Fahrenheit (35° Celsius) and 115° Fahrenheit (46° Celsius) for 4 - 6 hours.

HANDY TOOLS: large shallow glass dish and dehydrator.

Buttery Herb Pasta

INGREDIENTS:

- Buttery Italian Sauce (see page 55)
- 3 cups spiralized zucchini (see page 84)

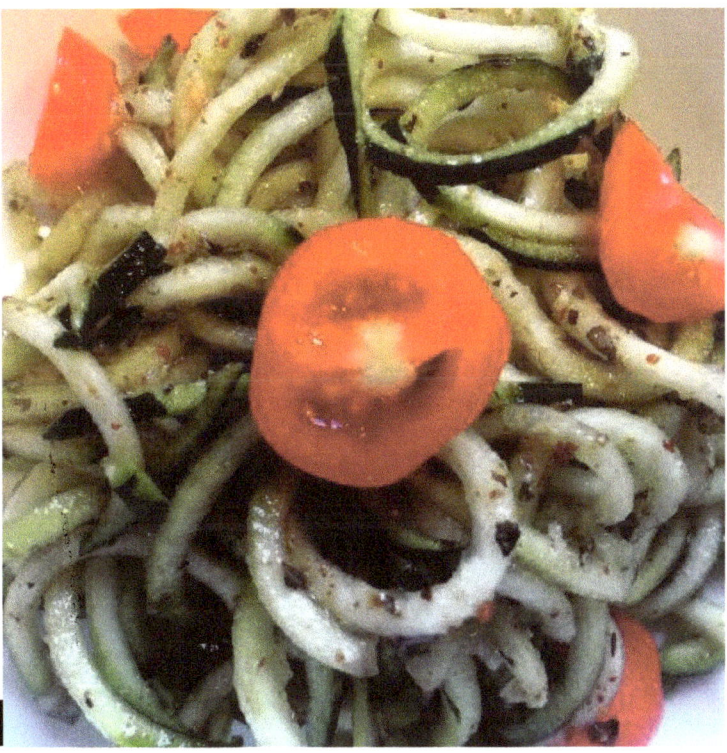

Photo Credit: TableTop Photography, Inc.

DIRECTIONS: Stir all of the buttery Italian sauce ingredients until well combined and then pour over spiralized zucchini. Stir well to coat. Optional, add chopped cherry tomatoes.

HANDY TOOLS: medium size bowl and a spiralizer.

eat! easy everyday raw vegan recipes!

Fish Cakes

INGREDIENTS:

- 1/2 cup sprouted dehydrated walnuts (see page 117)
- 1/2 cup sprouted dehydrated pecans (see page 117)
- 1/4 cup chopped red onion
- 1 Tbsp lime juice
- 1/2 Tbsp and 1/2 tsp kelp powder
- 1 tsp Celtic sea salt
- 1/2 tsp dill
- 1/2 tsp chili powder
- 1/4 tsp basil

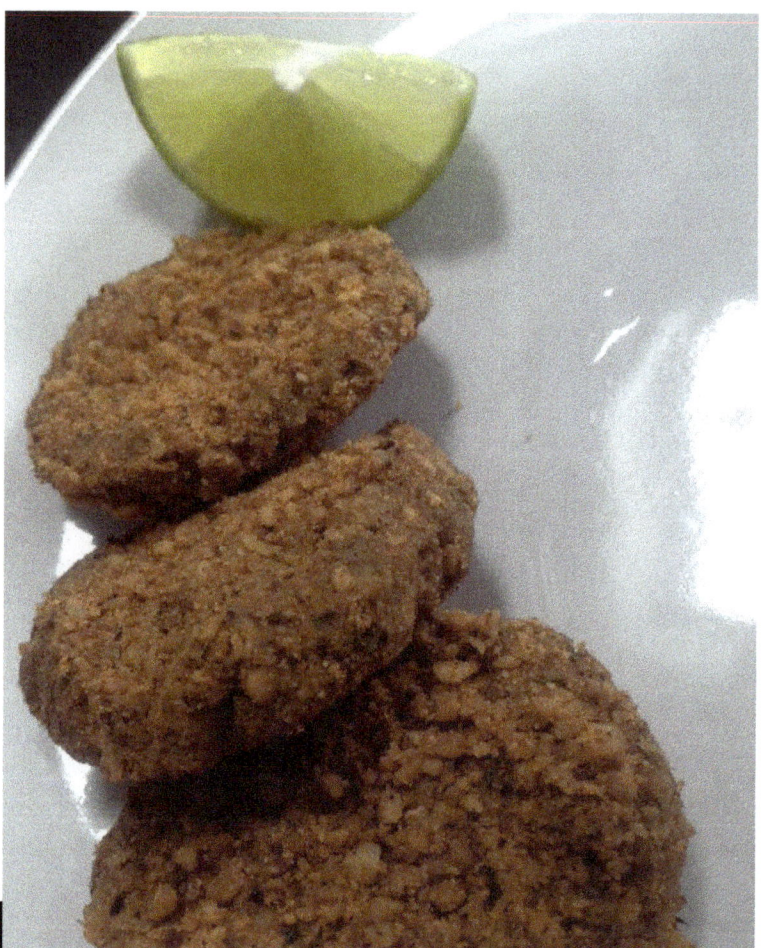

Photo Credit: TableTop Photography, Inc.

DIRECTIONS: blend walnuts and pecans together into a crumble using a food processor. Blend in remaining ingredients. Spoon into patties. Optional, reserve some of the blended walnut and pecan crumble to make a crust. Dehydrate between 95° Fahrenheit (35° Celsius) and 115° Fahrenheit (46° Celsius) for 8 hours, 4 hours on each side.

HANDY TOOLS: food processor.

Herb Turkey Slices

INGREDIENTS:

- 2 large portobello mushrooms
- 1/4 cup water
- 2 Tbsp olive oil
- 1 tsp sage
- 1 tsp onion powder
- 1 tsp thyme
- 1 tsp marjoram
- 1/2 tsp Celtic sea salt

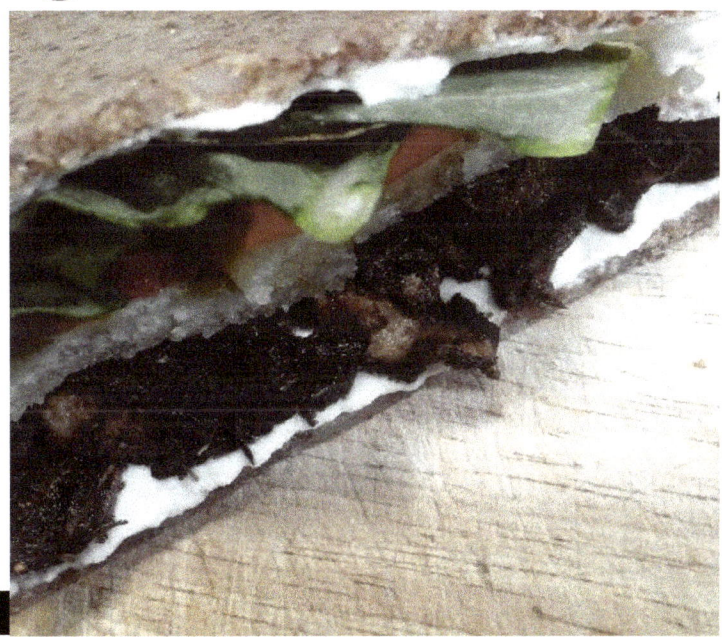

Photo Credit: TableTop Photography, Inc.

DIRECTIONS: slice mushrooms into strips or preferred size. Place all other ingredients together in a medium shallow glass or ceramic dish and stir until well combined. Add mushrooms to dish and cover the dish with plastic wrap. Place dish in refrigerator to marinate the mushrooms for at least 2 hours, then dehydrate between 95° Fahrenheit (35° Celsius) and 115° Fahrenheit (46° Celsius) for 2 hours.

HANDY TOOLS: medium shallow glass dish and dehydrator.

Hummus & Kale Cups

INGREDIENTS:

- 2 medium size kale leaves
- 1/4 cup of sesame and scallion hummus (see page 64)
- 1/4 cup chopped Roma tomatoes
- 1/4 cup chopped avocado

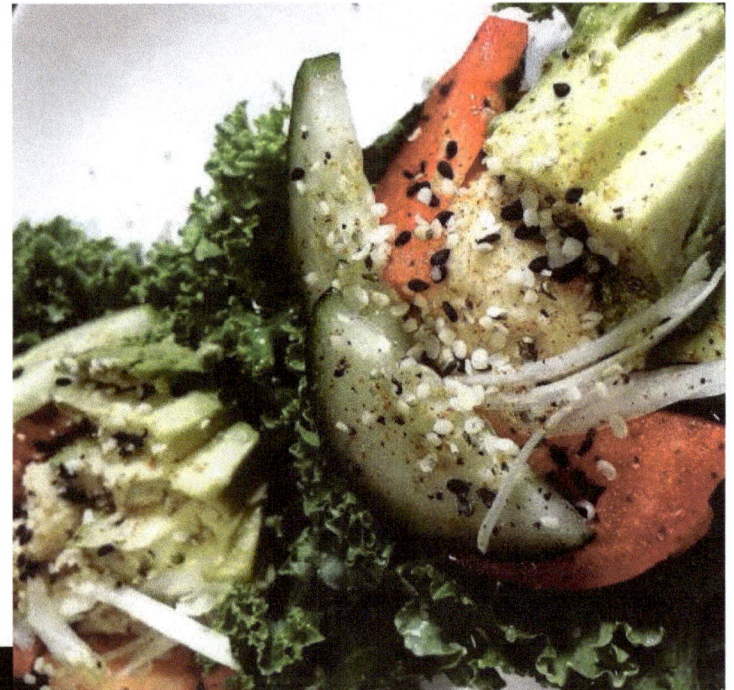

Photo Credit: TableTop Photography, Inc.

DIRECTIONS: fill each kale leaf with 2 Tbsp of the sesame and scallion hummus. Top with avocado and tomato. Optional, add thinly sliced yellow onions and sesame seeds.

HANDY TOOLS: (food processor for hummus, see page 64)

Jerk Seasoned Burger

INGREDIENTS:

- 2 cups sprouted, dehydrated walnuts (see page 117)
- 1 Tbsp jerk seasoning
- 1/2 tsp Celtic sea salt

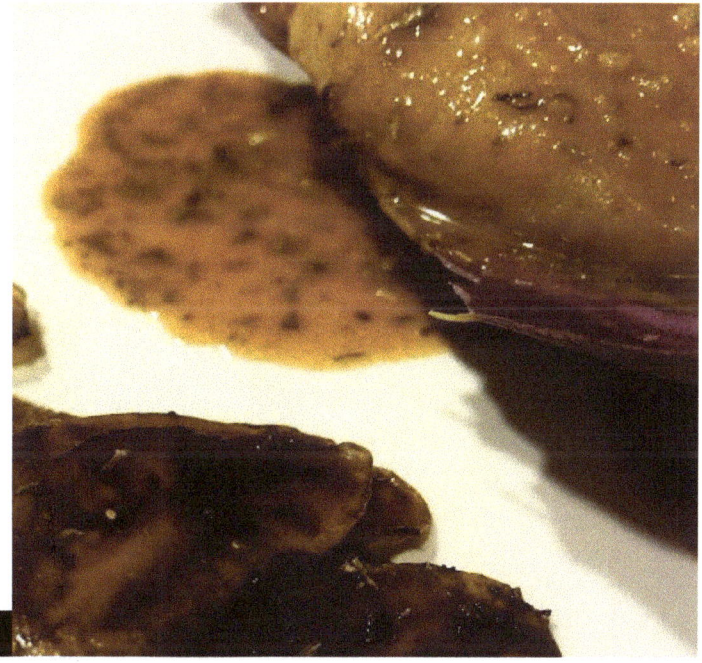

Photo Credit: TableTop Photography, Inc.

DIRECTIONS: blend all ingredients in a food processor then add 1 Tbsp of water. Shape into burger patties. Optional, drizzle on 1 Tbsp of unsalted jerk seasoned sauce (3 Tbsp of olive oil and 1 Tbsp of jerk seasoning).

HANDY TOOLS: food processor.

Jicama Herb Pizza Crust

INGREDIENTS:

- 1 cup chopped jicama
- 1/2 cup macadamia nuts
- 1/4 cup water
- 1/2 tsp oregano
- 1/4 tsp onion powder
- 1/4 tsp Celtic sea salt

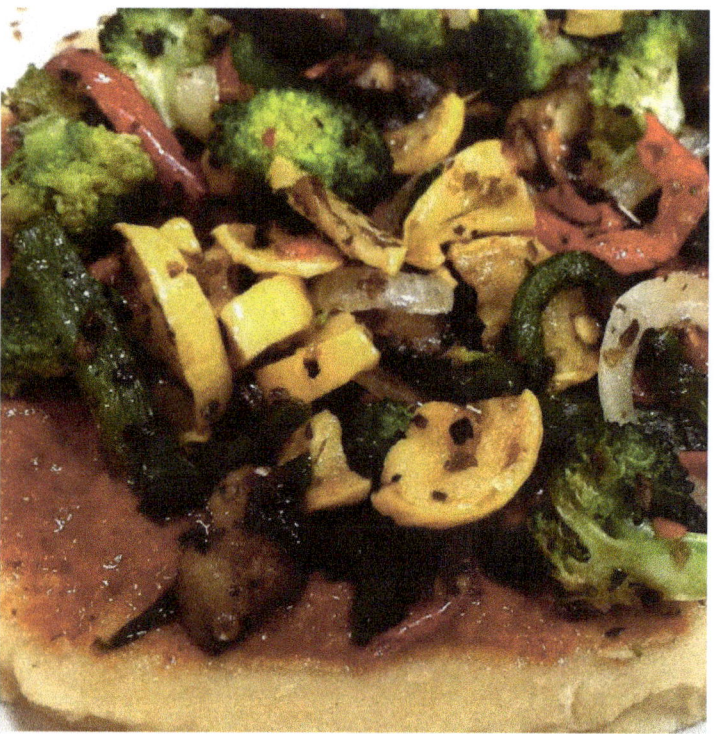

Photo Credit: TableTop Photography, Inc.

DIRECTIONS: blend ingredients until a dough forms. Dough will be slightly loose. Place the dough on a teflex sheet, shape into a 6 inch circle and dehydrate between 95° Fahrenheit (35° Celsius) and 115° Fahrenheit (46° Celsius) for 6 hours on each side.

HANDY TOOLS: blender and dehydrator.

eat! easy everyday raw vegan recipes!

Pesto Stuffed Mushrooms

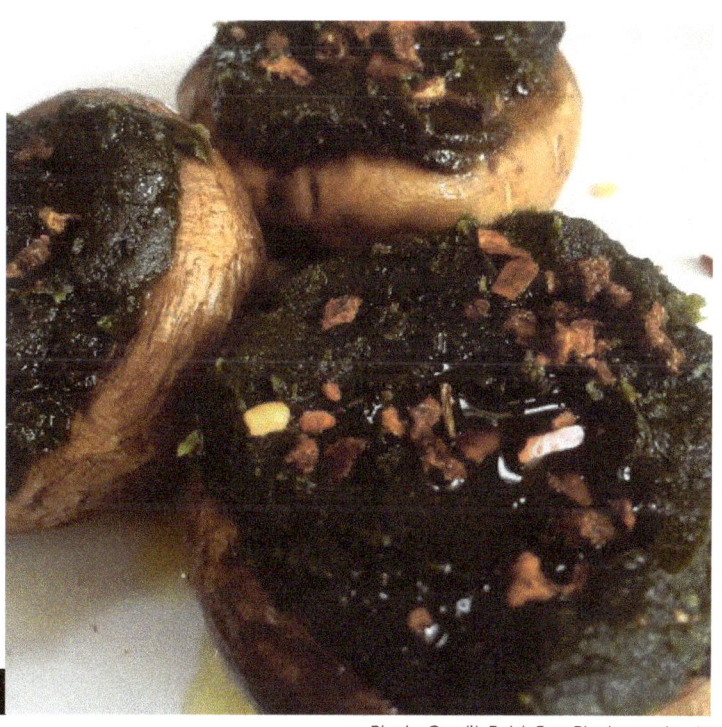

Photo Credit: TableTop Photography, Inc.

INGREDIENTS:

- 2 cups fresh basil
- 1 cup sprouted, dehydrated walnuts (see page 117)
- 1/2 cup macadamia nuts
- 1/3 cup olive oil
- 3 tsp onion powder
- 1/2 tsp Celtic sea salt
- 12 crimini mushroom caps

DIRECTIONS: place all ingredients (except mushroom caps) into food processor and blend until smooth. Then fill each mushroom cap with pesto mix. Place stuffed mushrooms on a teflex sheet and dehydrate between 95º Fahrenheit (35º Celsius) and 115º Fahrenheit (46º Celsius) for 8 hours.

HANDY TOOLS: dehydrator and medium size bowl.

eat! easy everyday raw vegan recipes!

Savory Pie Crust

INGREDIENTS:

- 1 cup sprouted, dehydrated walnuts (see page 117)
- 2 Tbsp chopped dates
- 1 Tbsp olive oil
- 1/2 tsp onion powder
- 1/2 tsp oregano
- 1/4 tsp Celtic sea salt

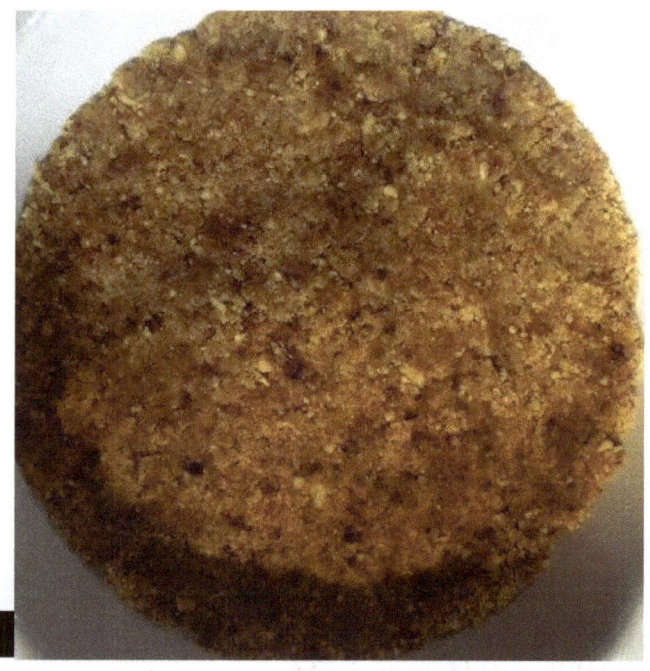

Photo Credit: TableTop Photography, Inc.

DIRECTIONS: place ingredients in a food processor. Blend until the ingredients form a ball, then press the ball into a pie dish. Use for your favorite savory pie filling.

HANDY TOOLS: food processor and pie dish.

Savory Vegetables

INGREDIENTS:

- 4 cups of assorted chopped vegetables (zucchini, summer squash, broccoli, peppers, cabbage)
- 1/3 cup water
- 3 Tbsp olive oil
- 2 Tbsp onion powder
- 1 tsp thyme
- 1/4 tsp Celtic sea salt
- Pinch of cayenne pepper (optional)

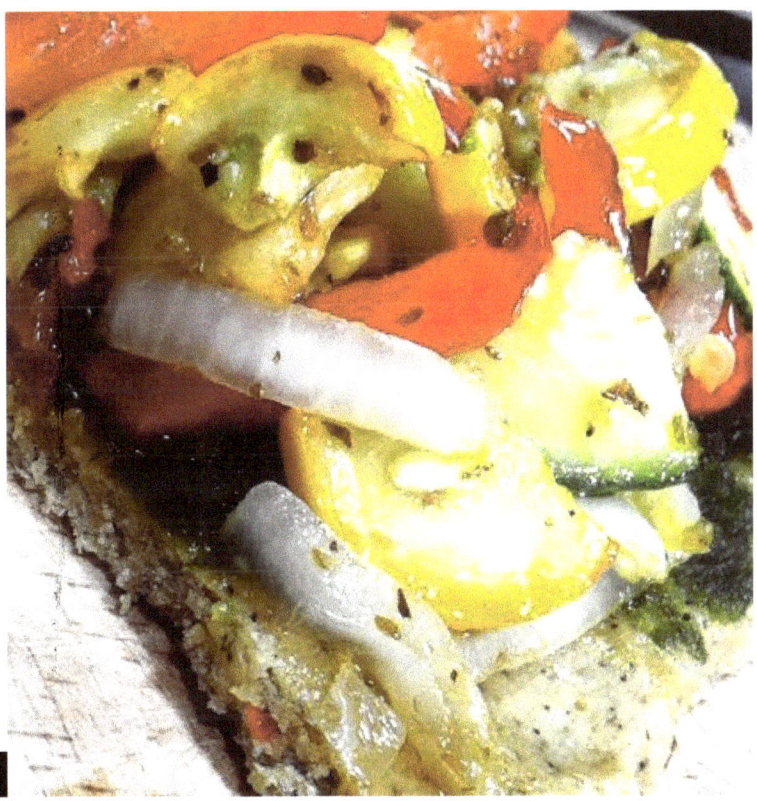

Photo Credit: TableTop Photography, Inc.

DIRECTIONS: place all ingredients in a large shallow glass dish and stir until well combined. Dehydrate between 95° Fahrenheit (35° Celsius) and 115° Fahrenheit (46° Celsius) for 4 - 6 hours.

HANDY TOOLS: large shallow glass dish and dehydrator.

Spicy Meatballs

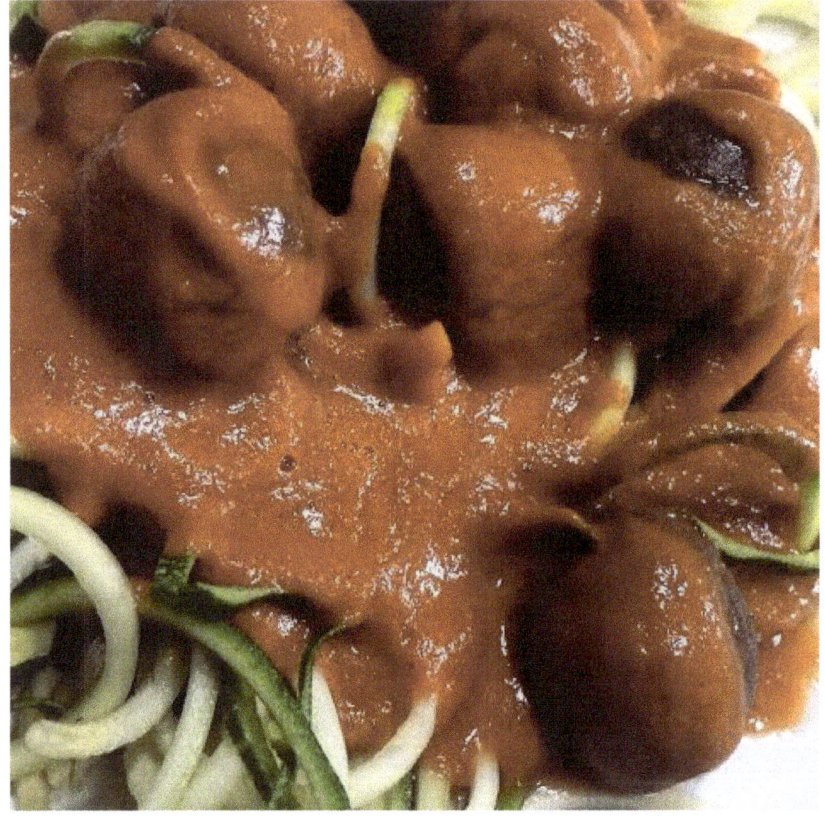

Photo Credit: TableTop Photography, Inc.

INGREDIENTS:

- 3 cups sprouted, dehydrated walnuts (see page 117)
- 1/4 chopped onion
- 2 Tbsp olive oil
- 2 Tbsp chopped dates
- 1 Tbsp oregano
- 1 Tbsp sage
- 2 tsp thyme
- 1 tsp crushed red pepper flakes
- 1 tsp Celtic sea salt

DIRECTIONS:
place all ingredients in a food processor and blend until well combined. Shape into "meatballs" and place on teflex sheet. Dehydrate between 95° Fahrenheit (35° Celsius) and 115° Fahrenheit (46° Celsius) for 2 - 4 hours.

HANDY TOOLS:
dehydrator and food processor.

Taco Crumble

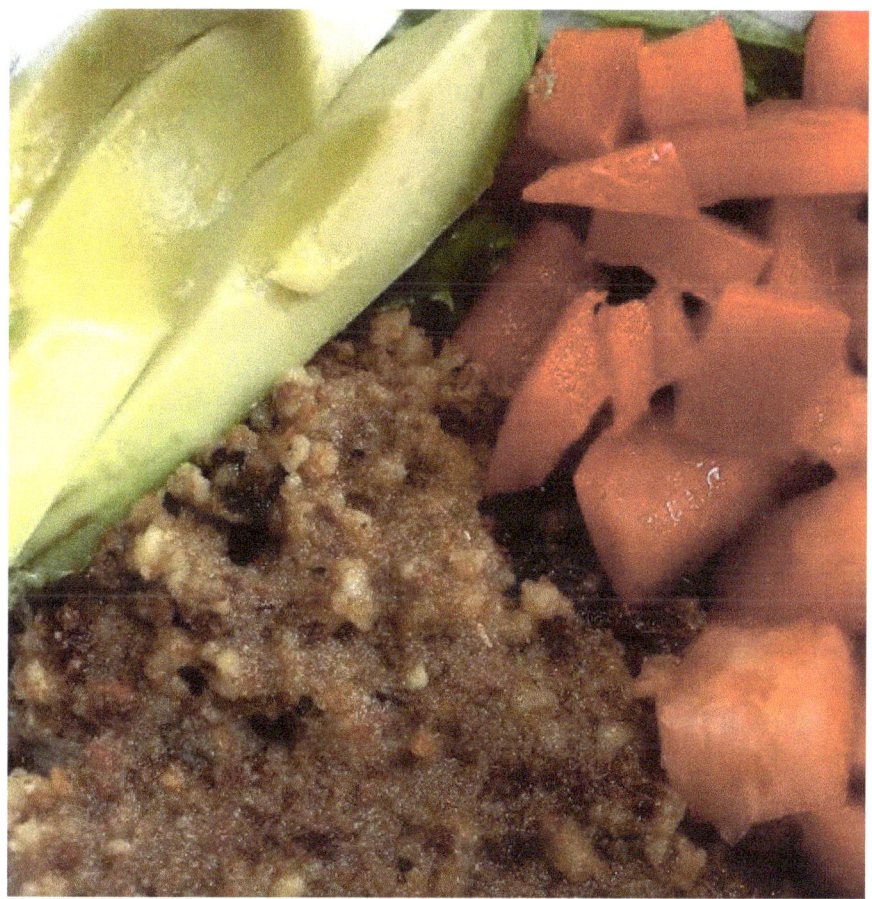

Photo Credit: TableTop Photography, Inc.

INGREDIENTS:

- 1 cup sprouted, dehydrated walnuts (see page 117)
- 1 Tbsp cumin
- 1 tsp chili powder
- 1/2 tsp Celtic sea salt

DIRECTIONS: place all ingredients in a food processor and blend until the walnuts are completely crumbled.

HANDY TOOLS: food processor.

eat! easy everyday raw vegan recipes!

Vegetable Pot Pie

INGREDIENTS:

Cream Sauce
- 1 and 1/2 cups water (add additional 1/4 cup of water if sauce is not 'loose' enough)
- 1 cup macadamia nuts
- 1 Tbsp dill
- 1 tsp Celtic sea salt
- 1 tsp onion powder
- Savory Pie Crust (see page 78)

Vegetables
- 2 cups assorted chopped fresh vegetables (zucchini, broccoli, peppers, etc.)

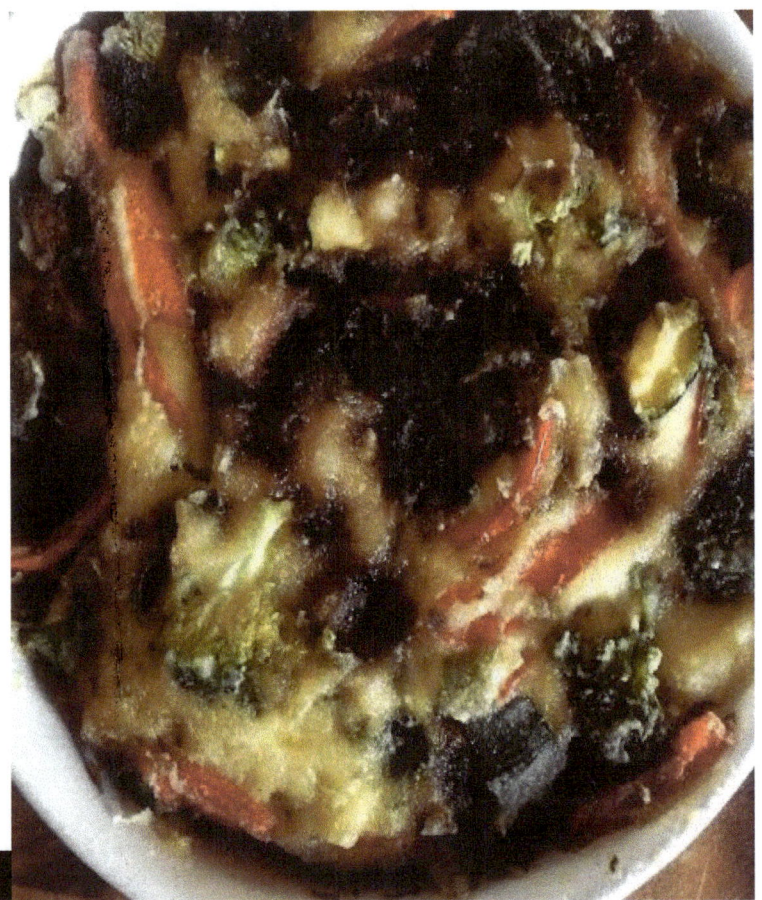

Photo Credit: TableTop Photography, Inc.

DIRECTIONS: add all cream sauce ingredients (except dill) to a food processor and blend until completely smooth. Then add chopped vegetables to a medium size bowl and pour your cream sauce mixture over the vegetables, add dill and stir until the vegetables are well coated. Place the coated vegetables in the savory pie crust (see page 78) and dehydrate between 95° Fahrenheit (35° Celsius) and 115° Fahrenheit (46° Celsius) for 8 hours.

HANDY TOOLS: dehydrator, food processor, and

Walnut "Turkey" Burgers

INGREDIENTS:

- 2 cups sprouted walnuts (see page 117)
- 2 Tbsp olive oil
- 1 Tbsp water
- 1 Tbsp sage
- 1 tsp marjoram
- 1/2 tsp onion powder
- 1/2 tsp oregano
- 1/4 tsp Celtic sea salt
- 1/4 tsp of crushed red pepper flakes

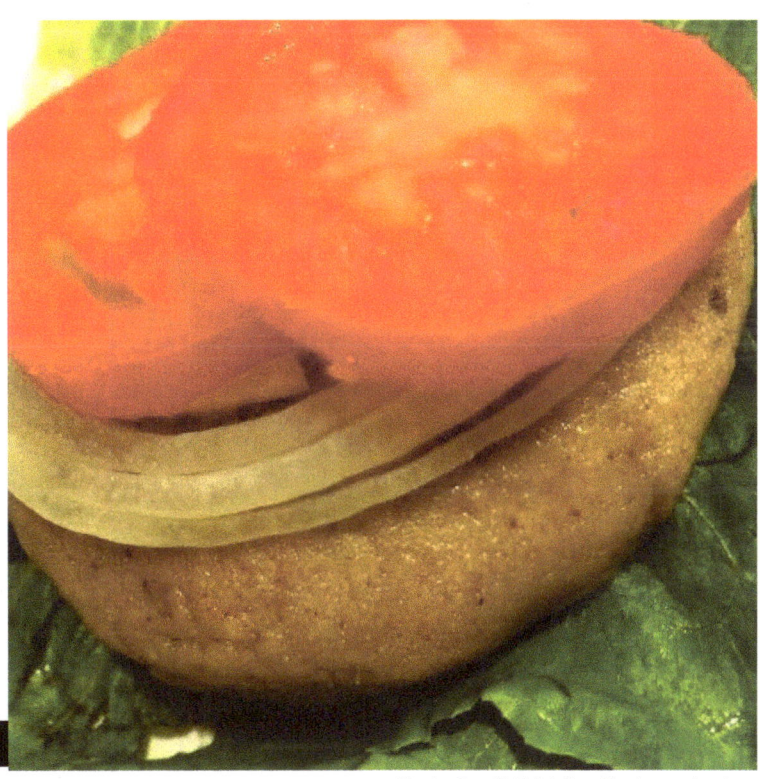

Photo Credit: TableTop Photography, Inc.

DIRECTIONS: blend all ingredients in a blender until well combined. Form into two equal sized burger patties. Set in fridge overnight to firm or serve immediately.

HANDY TOOLS: food processor.

Zucchini Noodles

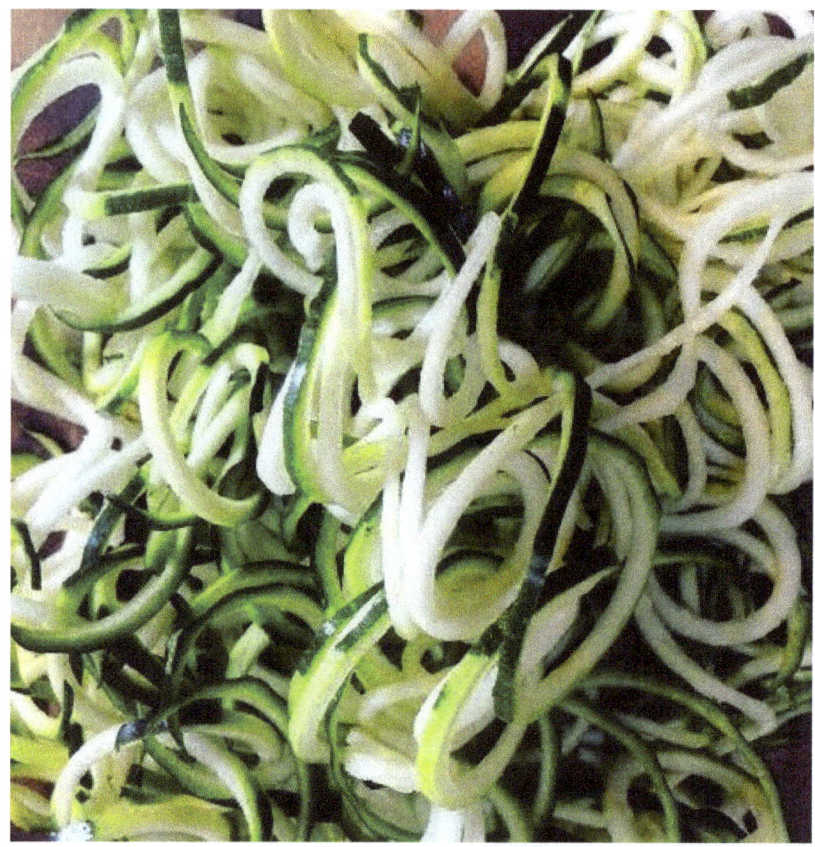

Photo Credit: TableTop Photography, Inc.

INGREDIENTS:

- 2 medium size courgettes (zucchini)

DIRECTIONS:
use a spiralizer (see page 117) to create a noodle shape from the courgettes. Top with your favorite raw vegan pasta sauce.

HANDY TOOLS:
spiralizer.

Sides

Caramelized Onions

INGREDIENTS:

- 1 cup thin sliced yellow onions
- 1/2 cup water
- 1/4 cup date paste (see page 43)
- 1 Tbsp olive oil
- 1/4 tsp Celtic sea salt

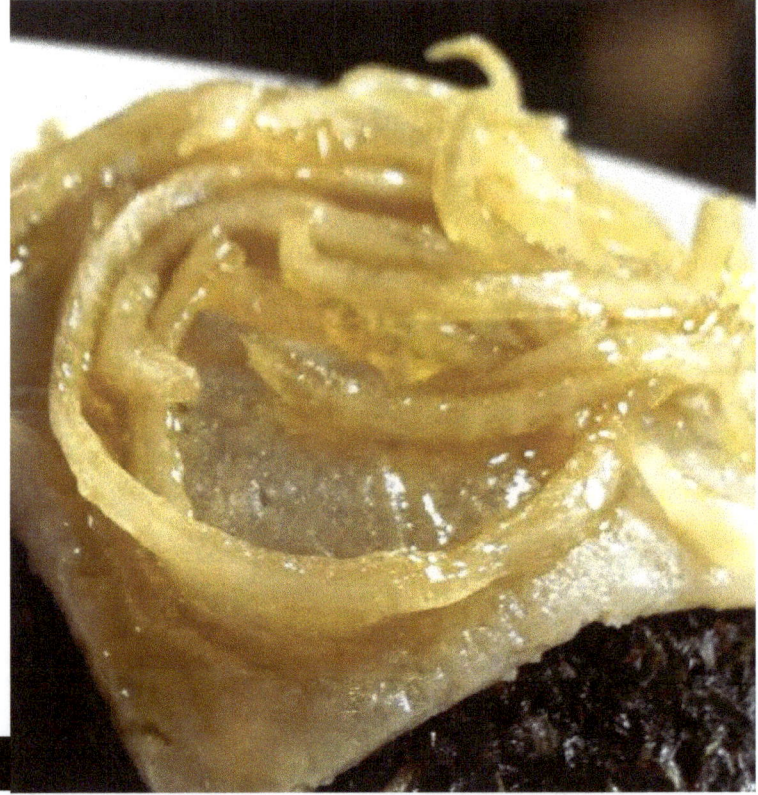

Photo Credit: TableTop Photography, Inc.

DIRECTIONS: place all ingredients in a medium bowl and stir until well combined. Spread coated onion slices on a teflex sheet and dehydrate between 95° Fahrenheit (35° Celsius) and 115° Fahrenheit (46° Celsius) for 3 hours.

HANDY TOOLS: dehydrator and medium size bowl.

eat! easy everyday raw vegan recipes!

Coconut Rice

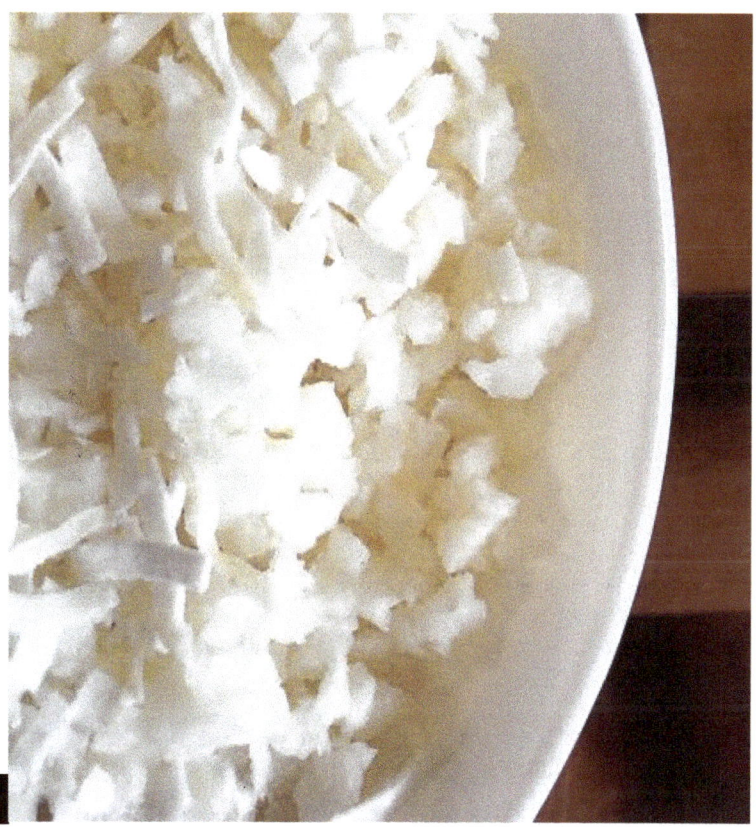

INGREDIENTS:

- 1 cup peeled and chopped jicama
- 1/4 cup coconut shreds
- 1 Tbsp coconut oil
- 1/2 tsp thyme
- 1/4 tsp onion powder
- 1/4 - 1/2 tsp Celtic sea salt (to taste)

Photo Credit: TableTop Photography, Inc.

DIRECTIONS: place all ingredients together in a food processor and process until the jicima takes on a "rice like" appearance.

HANDY TOOLS: food processor.

Creamed Broccoli

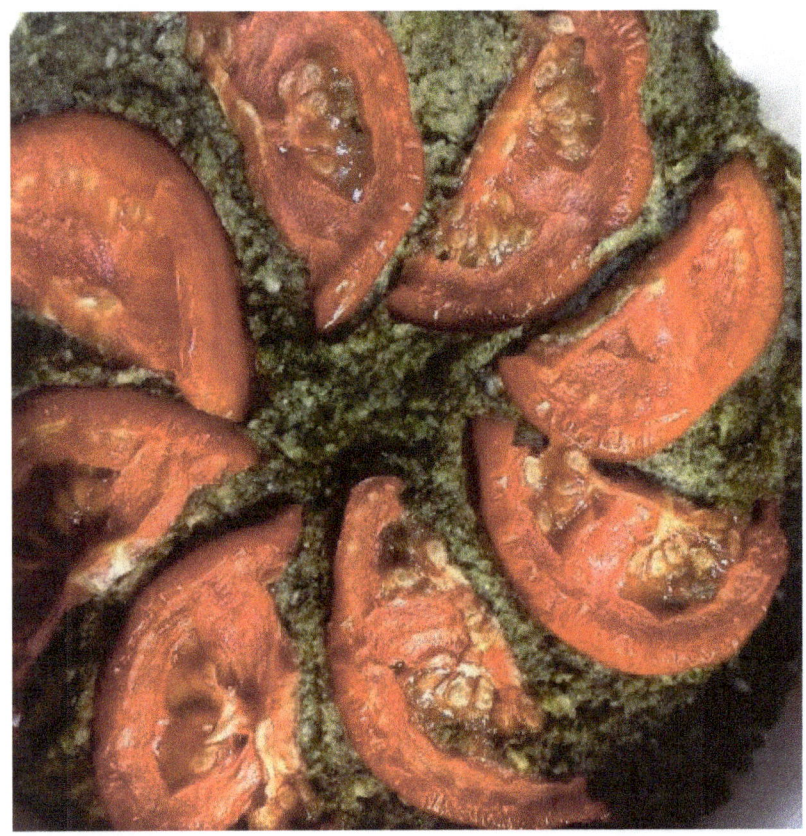

Photo Credit: TableTop Photography, Inc.

INGREDIENTS:

- 2 and 1/2 cups broccoli florets
- 1/2 cup macadamia nuts
- 3 Tbsp olive oil
- 1 tsp onion powder
- 1/2 tsp Celtic sea salt

DIRECTIONS:
blend all ingredients together until smooth. Place in dehydrator between 95° Fahrenheit (35° Celsius) and 115° Fahrenheit (46° Celsius) for 2 hours.

HANDY TOOLS:
dehydrator and blender.

Crispy Mushrooms

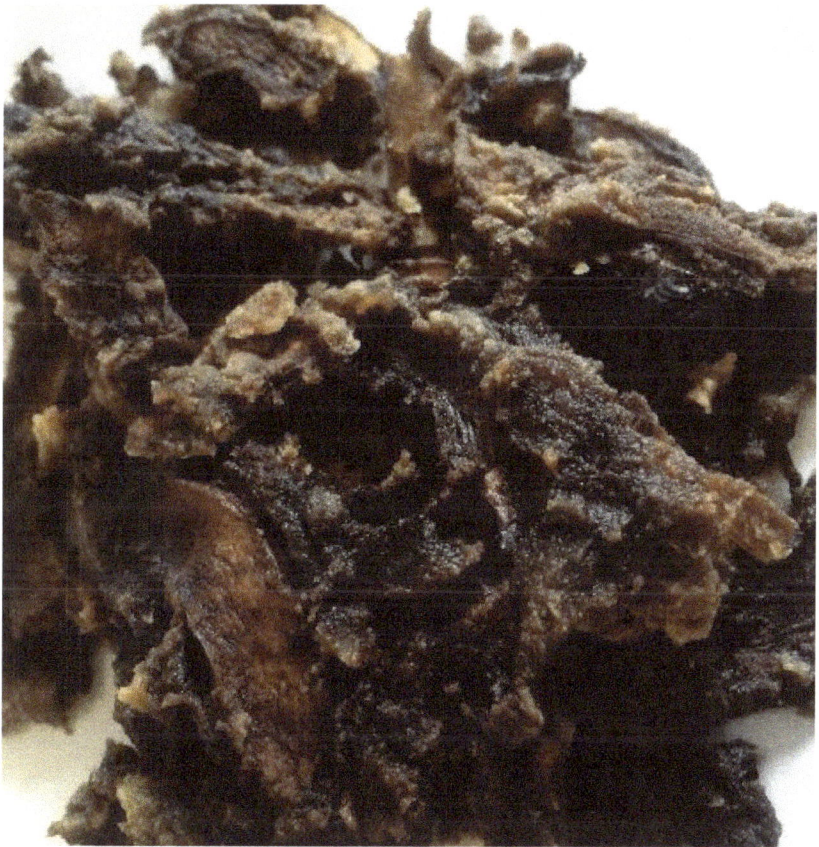

Photo Credit: TableTop Photography, Inc.

INGREDIENTS:

Cream Sauce
- 1/2 cup raw macadamia nuts
- 1/3 cup water
- 1/2 tsp chili seasoning mix
- 1/2 tsp Celtic sea salt
- 1/4 tsp thyme

Mushrooms
- 2 cups crimini mushrooms, thinly sliced

DIRECTIONS:
blend cream sauce ingredients until smooth. Pour over sliced mushrooms, stir until well coated, and dehydrate mushrooms between 95° Fahrenheit (35° Celsius) and 115° Fahrenheit (46° Celsius) on a teflex sheet for 12 - 15 hours.

HANDY TOOLS:
blender and dehydrator.

eat! easy everyday raw vegan recipes!

Fiesta Rice

INGREDIENTS:

- 4 cups of soaked bloomed wild rice (see page 113)
- 1 cup chopped Roma tomato
- 1/4 cup olive oil
- 2 Tbsp chopped cilantro
- 2 Tbsp chili powder
- 2 Tbsp onion powder
- 1 tsp cumin
- 1 tsp Celtic sea salt
- 1/4 tsp crushed red pepper flakes (optional)

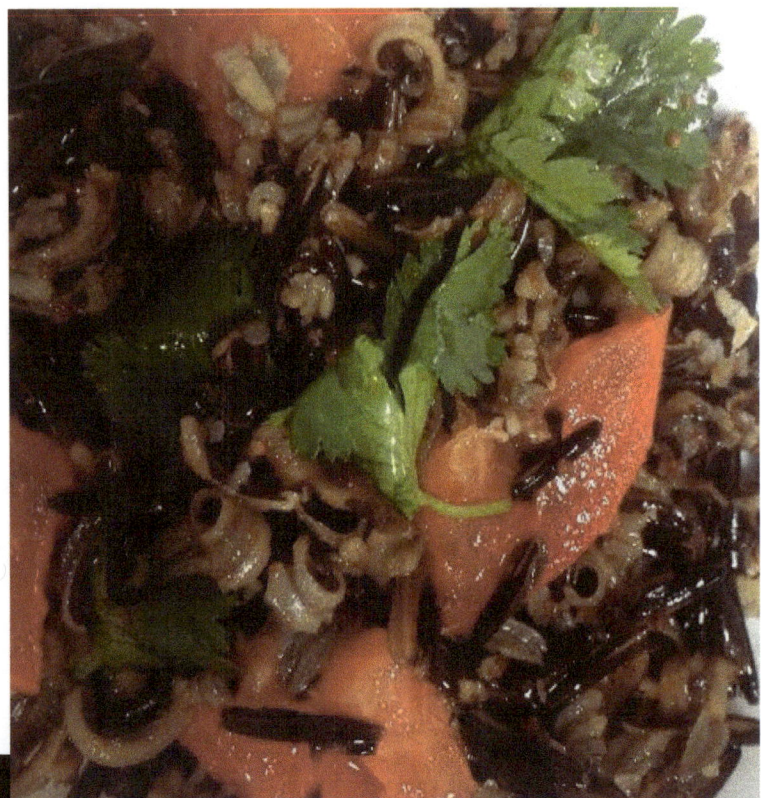

Photo Credit: TableTop Photography, Inc.

DIRECTIONS: place all ingredients (except Roma tomato and cilantro) together in a large bowl and stir thoroughly. Add in 1 cup of chopped Roma tomato and 2 Tbsp of chopped cilantro.

HANDY TOOLS: small bowl.

eat! easy everyday raw vegan recipes!

Jicama Rosemary Rice

INGREDIENTS:

- 2 cups peeled and chopped jicama
- 1/4 cup macadamia nuts
- 2 tsp raw agave or date paste (see page 43)
- 1 tsp dried rosemary
- 1/2 tsp onion powder
- 1/4 tsp Celtic sea salt

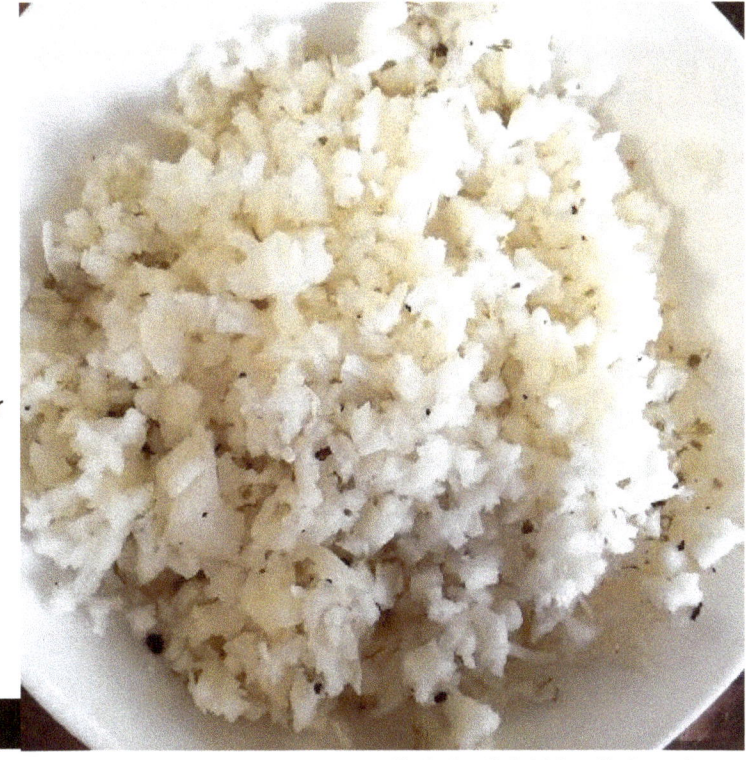

Photo Credit: TableTop Photography, Inc.

DIRECTIONS: place ingredients in food processor and pulse until jicama becomes "rice-like" in appearance.

HANDY TOOLS: food processor.

Kale & Cabbage Coleslaw

INGREDIENTS:

- 2 cups loosely packed chopped kale
- 2 cups loosely packed chopped cabbage
- 1/4 cup chopped onion
- 1/4 cup chopped red pepper
- 1/4 cup olive oil
- 1/4 cup apple cider vinegar
- 1/4 cup raw agave or date paste (see page 43)
- 1/4 tsp Celtic sea salt

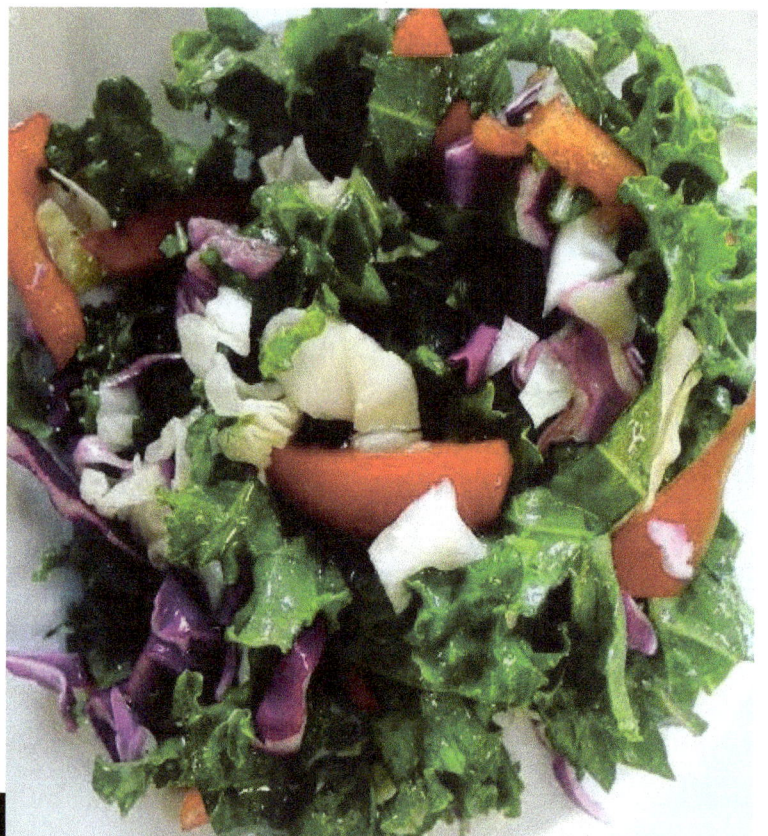

Photo Credit: TableTop Photography, Inc.

DIRECTIONS: place all ingredients in a large bowl and stir until well combined.

HANDY TOOLS: large bowl.

Marinated Cherry Tomatoes

INGREDIENTS:

- 1 cup cherry tomatoes, sliced in half
- 1/2 Tbsp olive oil
- 1/2 Tbsp raw agave or maple syrup (see page 116)
- 1/2 Tbsp apple cider vinegar
- 1/4 tsp oregano
- 1/8 tsp onion powder
- 1/8 tsp Celtic sea salt

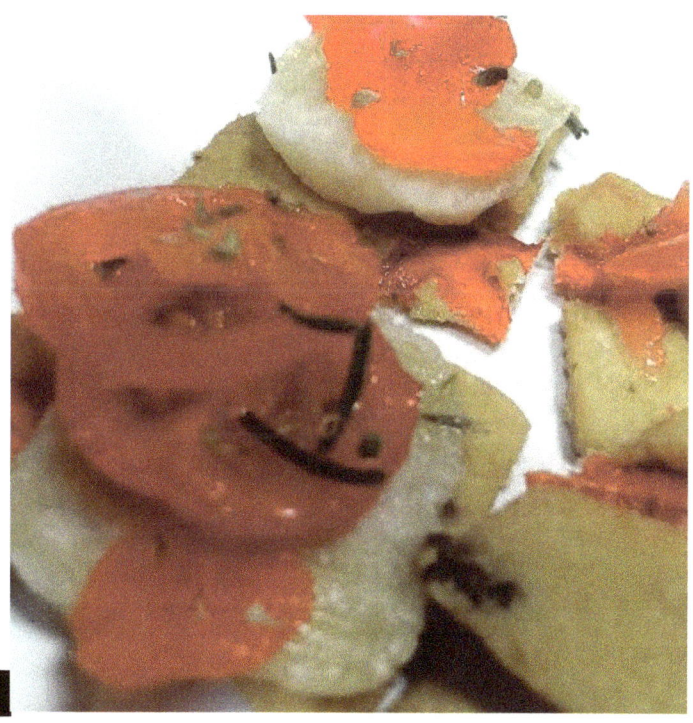

Photo Credit: TableTop Photography, Inc.

DIRECTIONS: place all ingredients in a medium size glass bowl and stir until well combined. Refrigerate overnight. Optional, dehydrate tomatoes between 95° Fahrenheit (35° Celsius) and 115° Fahrenheit (46° Celsius) for 1 - 2 hours.

HANDY TOOLS: medium size glass bowl.

Pickled Pink Onions

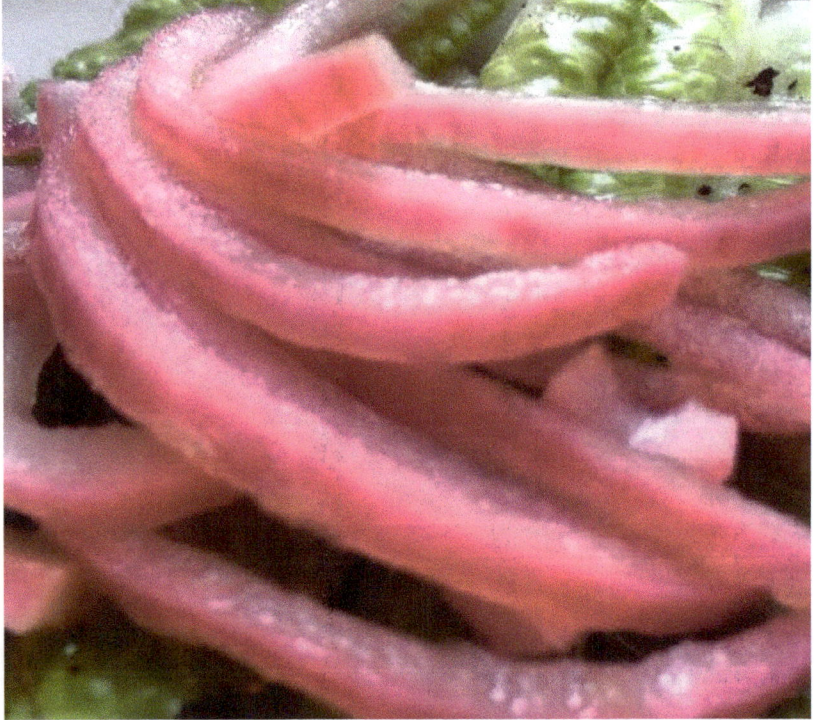

Photo Credit: TableTop Photography, Inc.

INGREDIENTS:

- 1/2 cup red onion, thinly sliced
- 1/4 cup apple cider vinegar
- 2 Tbsp olive oil
- 1/4 tsp Celtic sea salt

DIRECTIONS:
place all ingredients in shallow glass dish, stir until well combined. Marinate in refrigerator for 12 hours.

HANDY TOOLS:
shallow glass dish.

Sage Mashed Potatoes

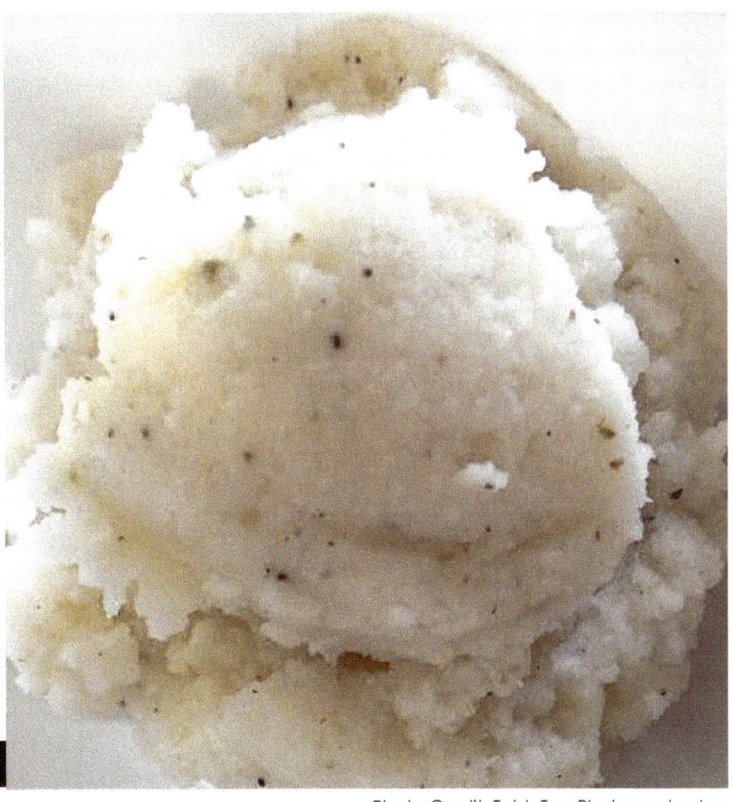

Photo Credit: TableTop Photography, Inc.

INGREDIENTS:

- 1 cup peeled and chopped jicama
- 1/2 cup macadamia nuts
- 1/4 cup water
- 1 tsp onion powder
- 1 tsp sage
- 1/2 tsp Celtic sea salt

DIRECTIONS: place all ingredients in a food processor and blend until smooth and creamy.

HANDY TOOLS: food processor.

eat! easy everyday raw vegan recipes!

Sesame Ginger Rice

INGREDIENTS:

- 2 cups bloomed wild rice (see page 113)
- 2 Tbsp sesame oil
- 1 tsp onion powder
- 1/2 tsp grated ginger
- 1/2 tsp Celtic sea salt

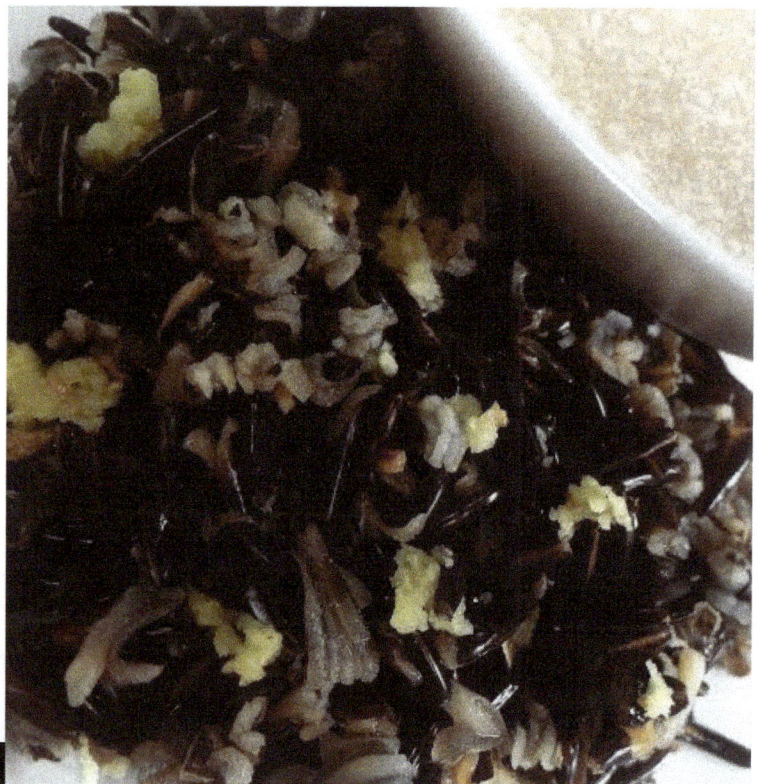

Photo Credit: TableTop Photography, Inc.

DIRECTIONS: place all ingredients together in a large bowl and stir until well combined.

HANDY TOOLS: large bowl and grater.

Sweet Sesame Wakame

INGREDIENTS:

- 1/2 cup of soaked and chopped wakame
- 1 tsp raw agave or date paste (see page 43)
- 1/2 tsp of sesame oil

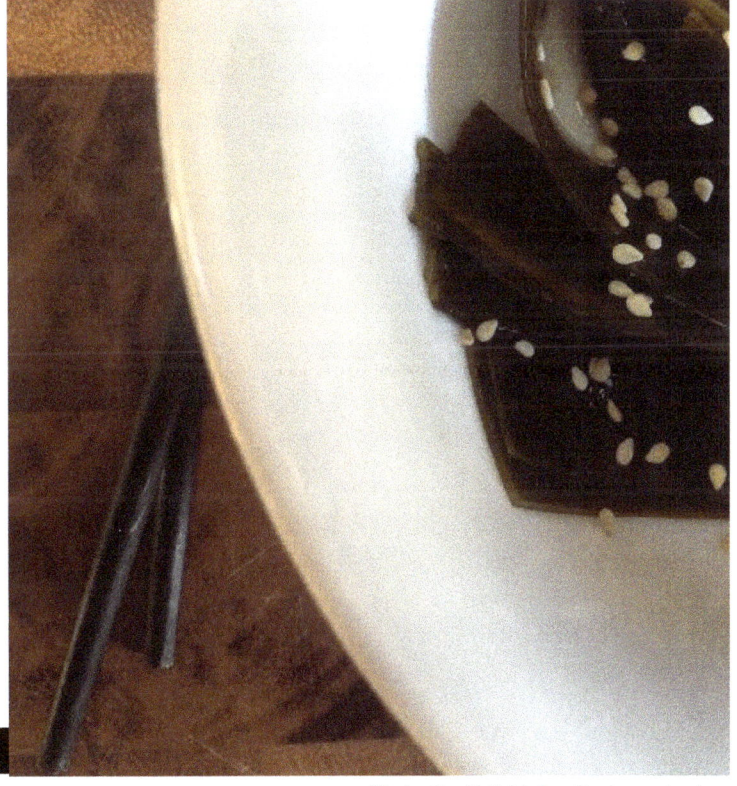

Photo Credit: TableTop Photography, Inc.

DIRECTIONS: place all ingredients in a bowl and stir thoroughly. Optional, garnish with sesame seeds.

HANDY TOOLS: small bowl.

eat! easy everyday raw vegan recipes!

Walnut & Apple Stuffing

INGREDIENTS:

- 1 cup sprouted walnuts (see page 117)
- 1 cup chopped crimini mushroom
- 1/2 cup finely chopped apple
- 2 Tbsp olive oil
- 2 Tbsp water
- 1/2 Tbsp oregano
- 1/2 Tbsp sage
- 1 tsp onion powder
- 1/2 tsp thyme
- 1/2 tsp Celtic sea salt

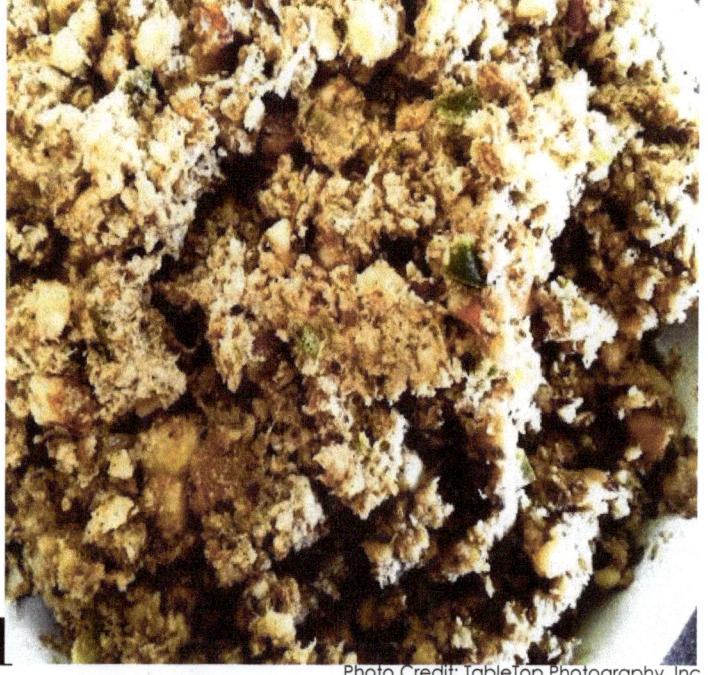

Photo Credit: TableTop Photography, Inc.

DIRECTIONS: blend nuts and spices together in a food processor and scoup into bowl. Add chopped mushrooms and chopped apples to bowl and stir until just combined. Then stir in olive oil and water. Optional add-in's: 1 Tbsp of finely chopped green pepper and 1/2 Tbsp of finely chopped yellow onion. Place in dehydrator between 95° Fahrenheit (35° Celsius) and 115° Fahrenheit (46° Celsius) for 2 hours.

HANDY TOOLS: dehydrator and food processor.

eat! easy everyday raw vegan recipes!

Wild & Spicy Plantains

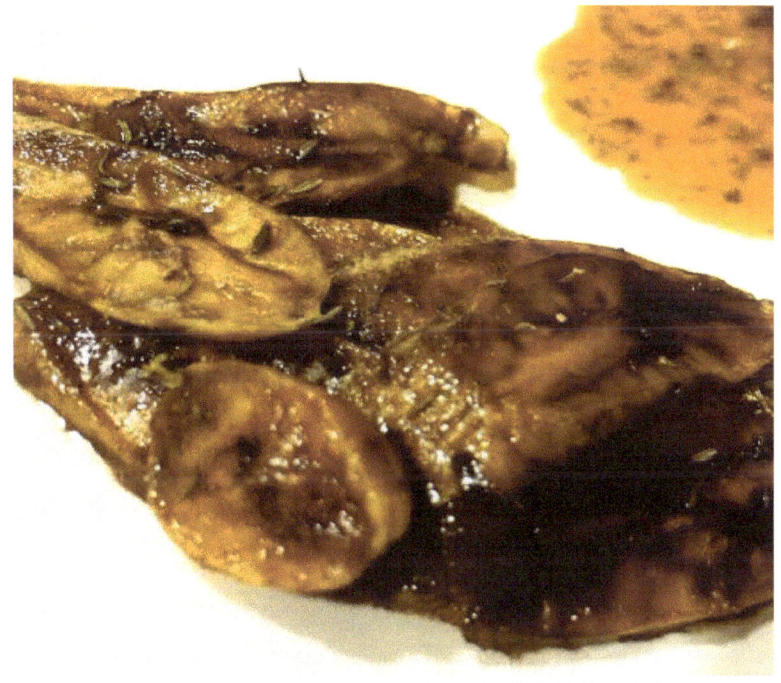

Photo Credit: TableTop Photography, Inc.

INGREDIENTS:

- 5 sliced baby bananas (see page 113)
- 1 Tbsp olive oil
- 1/2 tsp onion powder
- 1/4 tsp dried thyme
- 1/8 tsp Celtic sea salt

DIRECTIONS:
place all ingredients in a bowl and stir until well combined. Dehydrate the baby bananas between 95° Fahrenheit (35° Celsius) and 115° Fahrenheit (46° Celsius) for 8 hours.

HANDY TOOLS:
dehydrator and medium size bowl.

Wild Rice & Okra

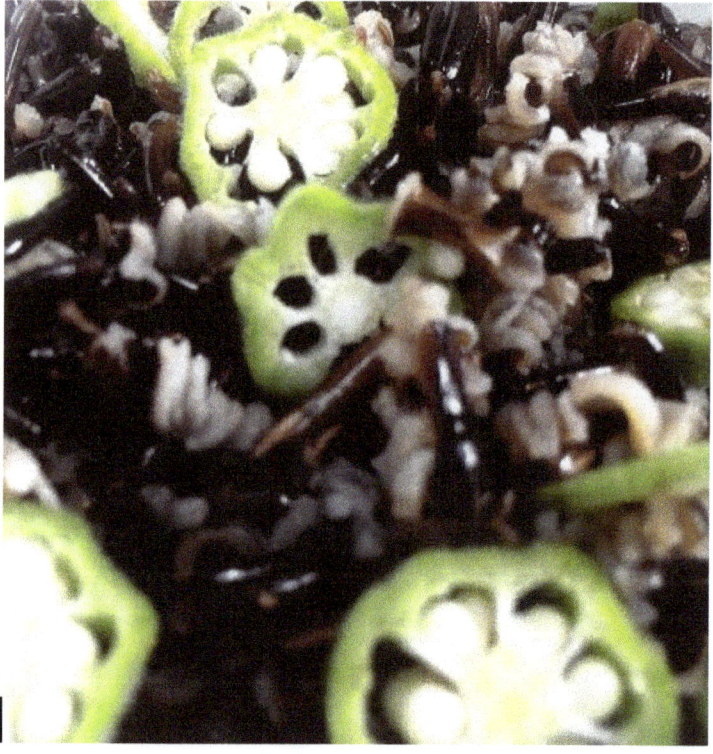

INGREDIENTS:

- 2 cups bloomed wild rice (see page 113)
- 1/2 cup thinly sliced okra
- 1/4 cup olive oil
- 2 Tbsp onion powder
- 1 Tbsp oregano
- 1 Tbsp marjoram
- 1 Tbsp Thyme
- 1 tsp Celtic sea salt

Photo Credit: TableTop Photography, Inc.

DIRECTIONS: place all ingredients in a large bowl and stir until well combined.

HANDY TOOLS: large size bowl.

Soups & Salads

Curry Squash Soup

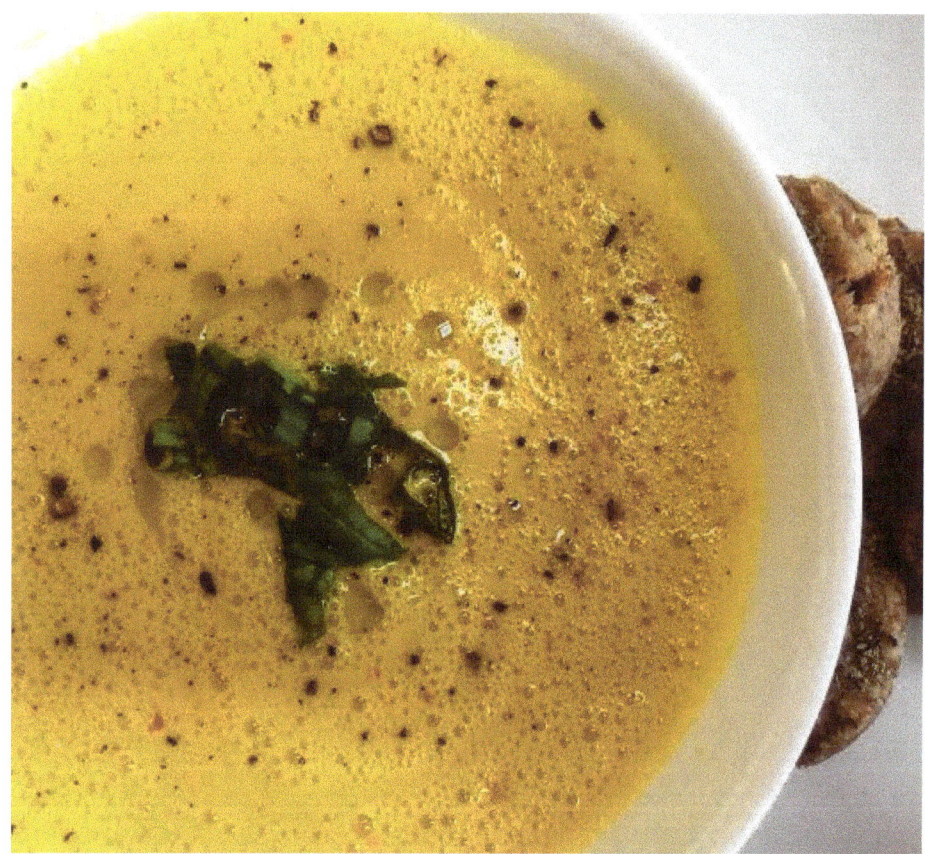

Photo Credit: TableTop Photography, Inc.

INGREDIENTS:

- 1 cup butternut squash
- 1 cup water
- 1 Tbsp coconut oil
- 1 Tbsp chopped dates
- 1/2 Tbsp curry powder
- 1 tsp onion powder
- 1/2 tsp Celtic sea salt

DIRECTIONS: place all ingredients in a food processor and blend until completely smooth.

HANDY TOOLS: food processor.

Fennel & Pear Gazpacho

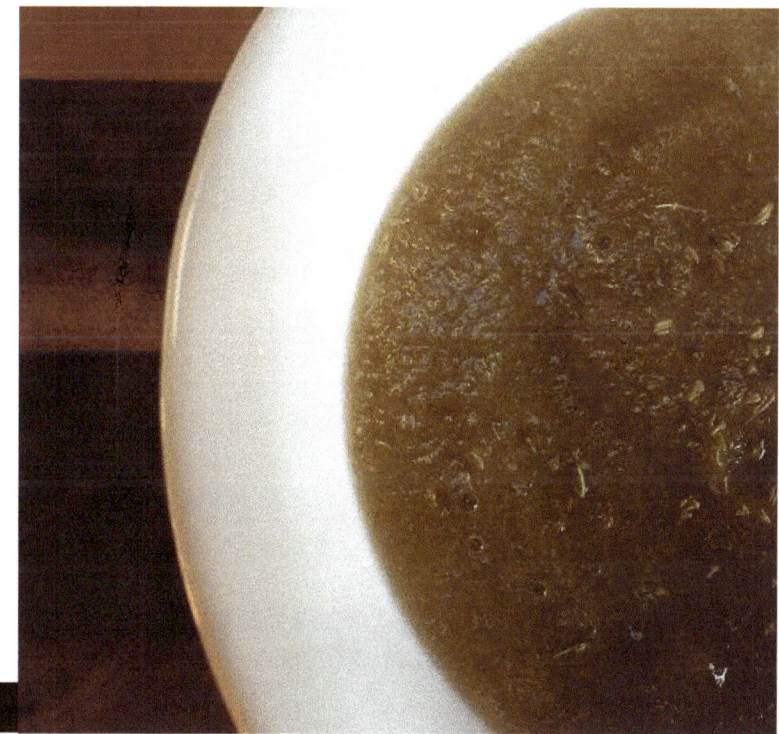

INGREDIENTS:

- 1 and 1/2 cups water
- 1 cup ripe green pear, peeled and chopped
- 1/2 cup chopped fresh fennel
- 1 Tbsp olive oil
- 1 Tbsp chopped dates
- 1 tsp onion powder
- 1 tsp Celtic sea salt

Photo Credit: TableTop Photography, Inc.

DIRECTIONS: place all ingredients in blender and blend until completely smooth.

HANDY TOOLS: blender.

Savory Zucchini Soup

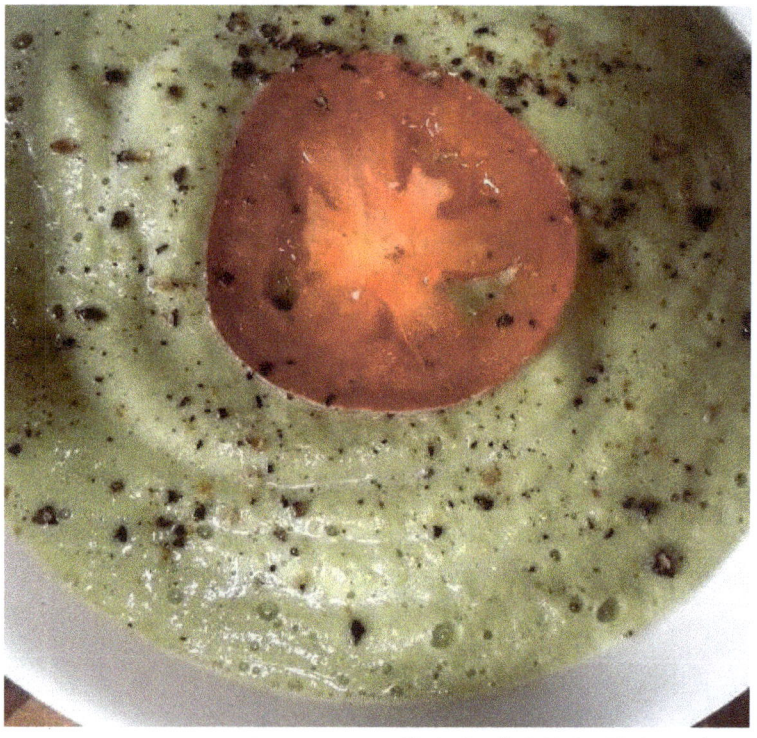

Photo Credit: TableTop Photography, Inc.

INGREDIENTS:

- 1 cup almond milk (see page 8)
- 1 cup chopped zucchini
- 1 avocado, chopped
- 1 Tbsp chopped onion
- 1/2 tsp Celtic sea salt

DIRECTIONS:
place all ingredients together in a blender and blend until completely smooth. Optional, add in chopped cherry or Roma tomato and/or red pepper.

HANDY TOOLS: blender.

eat! easy everyday raw vegan recipes!

Split Pea Soup

INGREDIENTS:

- 2 cups almond milk (see page 8)
- 1 cup chopped string beans
- 1/2 cup spinach (optional)
- 1/4 cup chopped onion
- 2 Tbsp avocado, chopped
- 2 Tbsp raw agave or date paste (see page 43)
- 1 tsp Celtic sea salt
- 1/2 tsp oregano

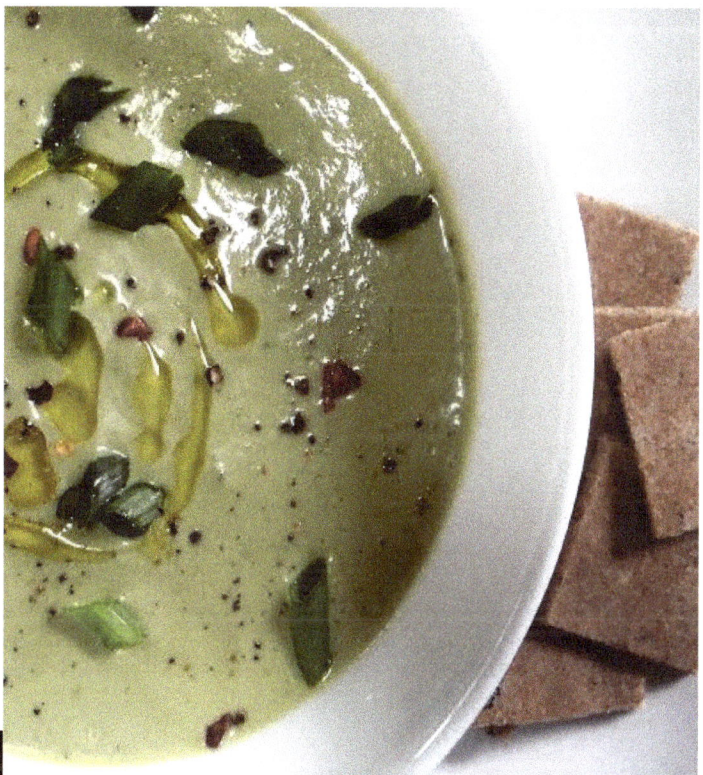

Photo Credit: TableTop Photography, Inc.

DIRECTIONS: place all ingredients in a blender and blend until well combined.

HANDY TOOLS: blender.

Sweet & Sour Soup

INGREDIENTS:

- 2 cups water (not heated above 105º Fahrenheit/ 40º Celsius)
- 1/4 cup chopped mushroom
- 3 Tbsp wakame flakes
- 2 Tbsp sesame oil
- 2 Tbsp date paste (see page 43)
- 2 Tbsp apple cider vinegar
- 1 tsp onion powder
- 1/2 tsp Celtic sea salt

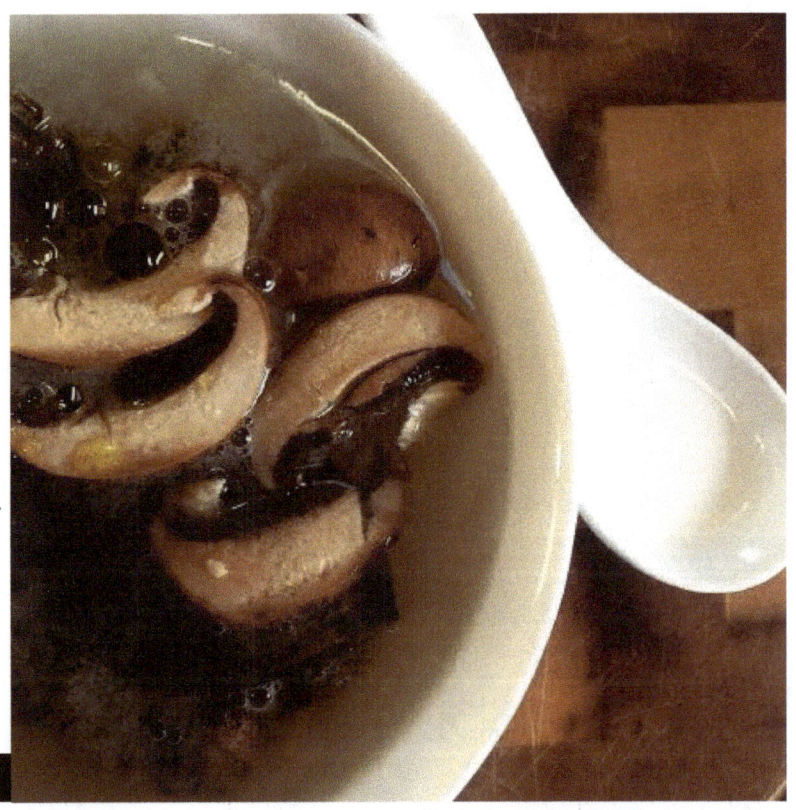

Photo Credit: TableTop Photography, Inc.

DIRECTIONS: add ingredients to a ready to serve (soup) bowl and stir. Optional, add thinly sliced yellow onion.

HANDY TOOLS: soup bowl.

Thai Coconut Soup

INGREDIENTS:

- 2 cups coconut milk (see page 13)
- 2 Tbsp chopped dates
- 1 Tbsp Thai seasoning
- 1 Tbsp lime juice
- 1 Tbsp olive oil
- 1 tsp Celtic sea salt
- 1 - 2 cups of finely chopped vegetables (red pepper, mushrooms, scallions)

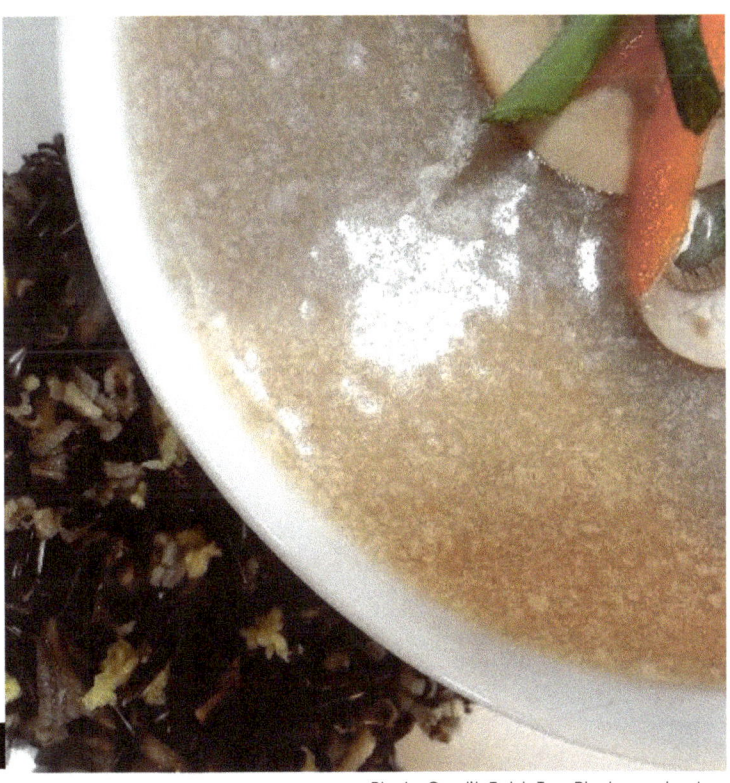

Photo Credit: TableTop Photography, Inc.

DIRECTIONS: blend all ingredients except finely chopped vegetables together in a blender until smooth. Pour over vegetables.

HANDY TOOLS: blender.

Autumn Pear Salad

INGREDIENTS:

- 2 cups romaine lettuce, chopped or shredded
- 1 cup sliced green pear
- 2 Tbsp olive oil
- 2 Tbsp raw agave or date paste (see page 43)
- 2 Tbsp apple cider vinegar
- 1/4 tsp Celtic sea salt

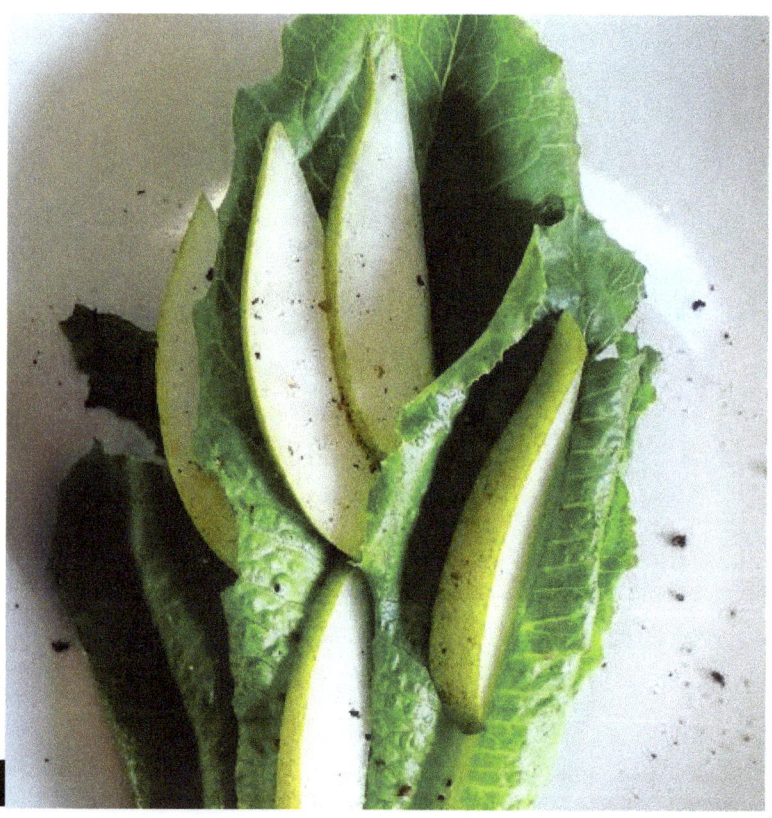

Photo Credit: TableTop Photography, Inc.

DIRECTIONS: place all ingredients in a large bowl and toss with tongs.

HANDY TOOLS: large size bowl and tongs.

eat! easy everyday raw vegan recipes!

Balsamic & Berry Fruit Salad

INGREDIENTS:

Berries
- 2 cups chopped strawberries
- 1 cup raspberries
- 1 cup blackberries
- 1/2 cup blueberries (optional)

Balsamic Vinegar Dressing
- 1/4 cup raw agave or maple syrup (see page 116)
- 2 Tbsp apple cider vinegar

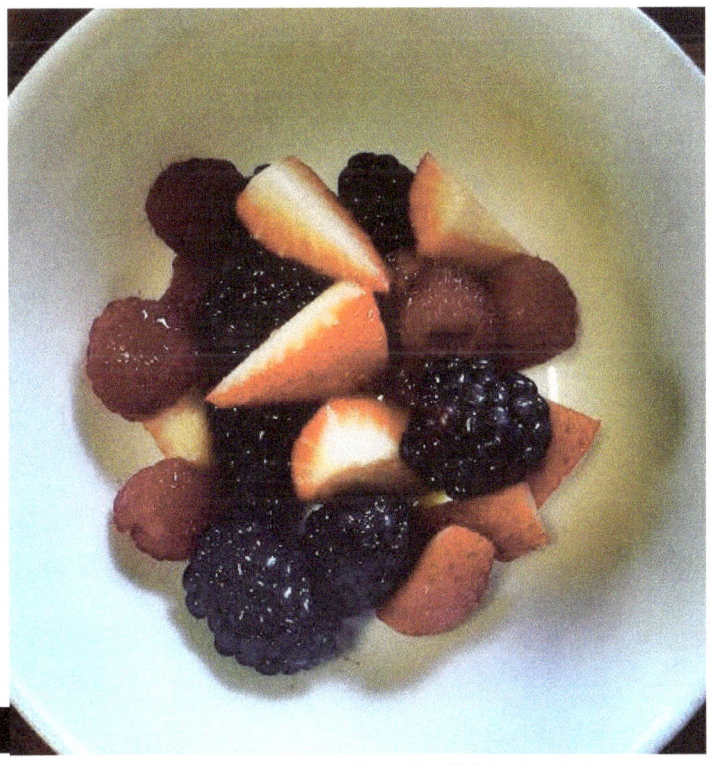

Photo Credit: TableTop Photography, Inc.

DIRECTIONS: place berries in medium size bowl and set to the side. Combine the balsamic vinegar dressing ingredients and pour over the berries. Stir until well combined.

HANDY TOOLS: medium size bowl.

Classic Garden Salad

INGREDIENTS:

- 2 cups shredded romaine or butter leaf lettuce
- 1 cup chopped cherry or Roma tomatoes
- 1/2 cup chopped cucumber
- 1/4 cup thinly sliced yellow onion
- 1/4 cup chopped avocado
- 2 Tbsp chopped raw olives (optional)

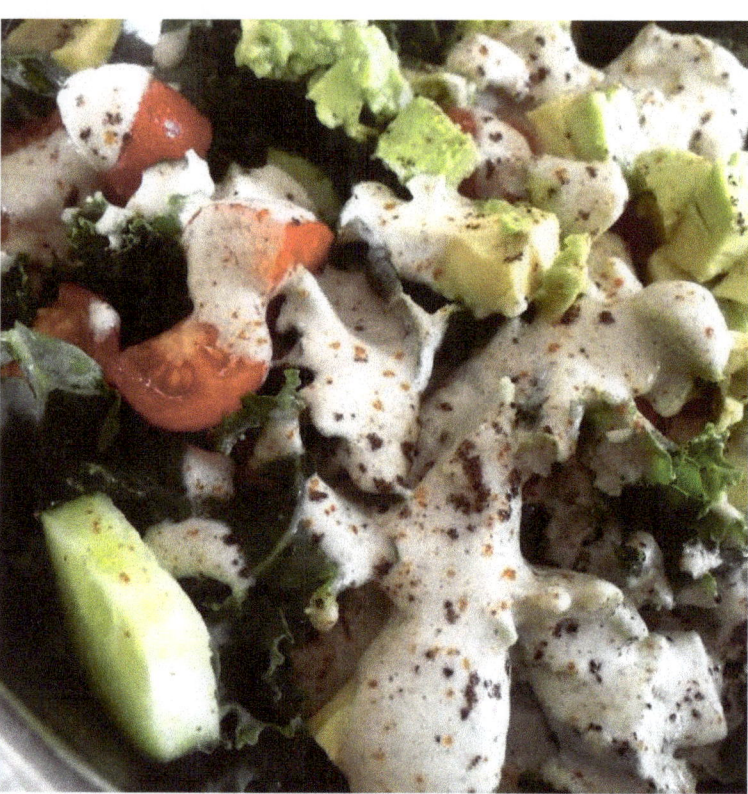

Photo Credit: TableTop Photography, Inc.

DIRECTIONS: place all ingredients in a large salad bowl and toss with olive oil and apple cider vinegar or your favorite raw vegan salad dressing.

HANDY TOOLS: large salad bowl and tongs.

Sea Veggie Salad

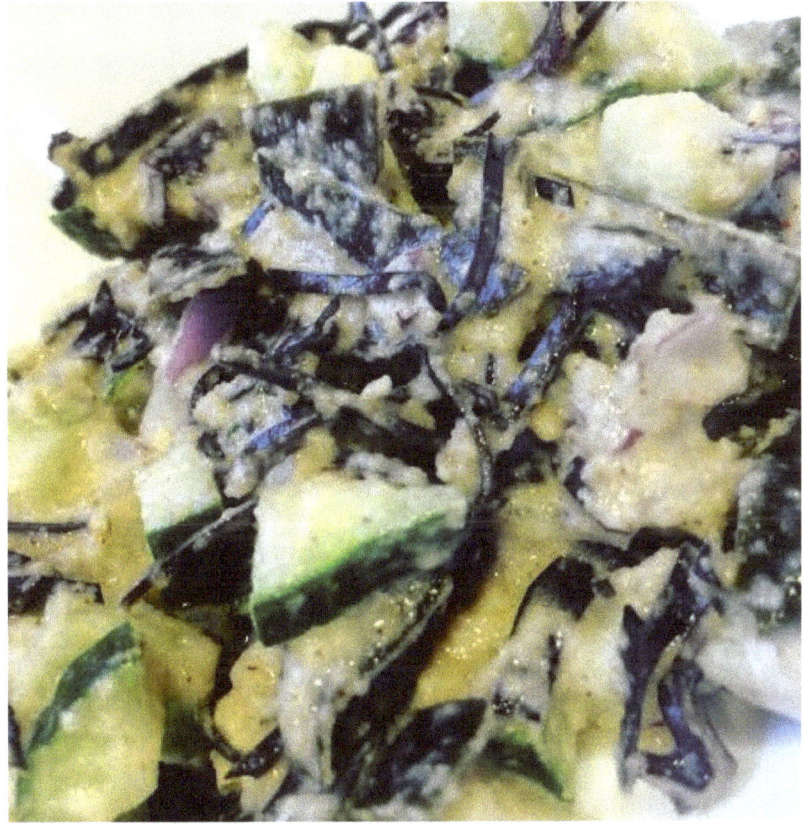

Photo Credit: TableTop Photography, Inc.

INGREDIENTS:

- 1/4 cup tahini dressing (see page 67)
- 1/4 cup chopped cucumbers
- 1/4 cup soaked wakame
- 2 Tbsp soaked arame
- 2 Tbsp chopped red onions

DIRECTIONS: stir all ingredients in a medium size glass bowl and serve chilled.

HANDY TOOLS: medium size glass bowl.

Raw Vegan Glossary

A

Almond Pulp (nut pulp) - almond pulp (or pulp from any nut) is the remaining part of the almonds after blending and straining soaked almonds to make almond milk.

Apple Cider Vinegar/ACV - apple cider vinegar, otherwise known as cider vinegar or ACV, is a type of raw vinegar made from apples and has a pale to medium amber color.

B

Baby Banana - a baby banana is a small, sweet variety of banana, one of the original species of banana before the "common household" bananas were genetically modified.

Bladderwrack - bladderwrack or fucus vesiculosus, known by the common name bladder wrack or bladderwrack, is a seaweed (sea vegetable). Most often used in the powder or flake form or after soaking the whole plant.

Bloomed - bloomed/bloom/blooming is a common term used for the process of sprouting wild rice. The end product is typically called "bloomed wild rice."

C

Carob Powder, Raw - raw carob powder is made from the long bean-like pods of the carob tree. Raw carob powder is used as a replacement for cacao or cocoa. It has a naturally sweet taste, without the stimulants typically found in chocolate. Raw carob powder is high in fiber, a good source of calcium, and has B vitamins, potassium and iron.

Coconut Flesh – coconut flesh is the edible tender fruit inside young Thai coconuts.

Cold-Pressed Extra Virgin Olive Oil - cold-pressed extra virgin olive oil, or sometimes referred to as Cold Pressed EVOO, is a raw cold-pressed olive oil made from raw olives.

Cold-Pressed Sesame Oil - cold-pressed sesame oil is a raw cold-pressed sesame oil made from raw sesame seeds.

Crimini Mushrooms - is an edible mushroom native to grasslands in Europe and North America. It has two color states while immature, white and brown.

Date Sugar - raw date sugar is actually dehydrated and ground dates. It can be used anywhere regular refined sugar is called for: cereal, baked goods, desserts, etc.

Dehydrator - a dehydrator is a tool that uses low temperatures and a fan to slowly dry food. It essentially removes the water from food, but at low temperatures, it keeps the enzymes of raw food intact.

Enzymes - enzymes are special proteins that act as the 'life force' in human beings. In both plants and animals, enzymes carry out all of the activities of metabolism. Enzymes from plants are retained when uncooked.

F

Foodism, Raw - raw foodism is the dietary practice of eating primarily uncooked, unprocessed foods.

Grapes, concord - concord grapes are a variety of grapes that are known to significantly boost the immune system and improve cardiovascular health. They have also been known to rid the body of excess mucus.

H

Heirloom - a traditional variety of plant (or breed of animal) that is not associated with large-scale commercial agriculture.

Honey, Raw - raw honey is honey (made by bees from flower nectar) that is pure, unheated, unpasteurized and unprocessed. *Note: Honey is not considered vegan by some.

I

Immune System - the immune system is the body's defense against infectious bacteria and other invaders. Through a series of steps called the immune response, the immune system attacks foreign substances that invade body systems and cause disease.

J

Jicama - jicama or Mexican yam bean, or Mexican turnip, is the name of a native Mexican vine, although the name most commonly refers to the plant's edible tuberous root.

Julienne - a portion of food cut into short, thin strips; the action of cutting food into short thin strips.

K

Kelp - kelp is seaweed (sea vegetable) that typically has a long, tough stalk with a broad frond divided into strips. It is most widely available in a dehydrated and powder form.

L

Leafy Greens - leafy greens are plant leaves eaten as a vegetable.

Lucuma Powder - Lucuma powder is made from whole Peruvian lucuma fruit that has been dried at low temperatures and milled into a fine powder. Lucuma contains many nutrients including beta-carotene, iron, zinc, vitamin B3, calcium, and protein.

M

Maple Syrup, Grade B - Maple syrup is made from the sap of sugar maple, red maple, or/an black maple trees. Pure Grade B Maple Syrup is less refined than Grade A and contains many beneficial nutrients, including minerals such as potassium and iron. Note: maple syrup is not considered raw.

Marinate/Marinated - marinate/marinated is the action of soaking or food soaked in a liquid typically mixed with herbs and seasonings.

Marjoram - marjoram is an aromatic southern European plant of the mint family, the leaves of which are used as a culinary herb.

N

Non-GMO - the acronym GMO stands for Genetically Modified Organisms, which refers to any food product that has been altered at the gene level. Non-GMO foods **have not** been genetically altered in any way.

Non-hybrid - non-hybrid refers to seeds which have been naturally pollinated, also called open-pollinated.

Nori - nori is an edible seaweed (sea vegetable) eaten either fresh or dried in sheets.

O

Olives, Raw - olives that have been harvested from the tree but not yet cured and have been naturally sundried.

Organic - the term organic refers to produce and other foods that are grown without the use of pesticides, synthetic fertilizers, sewage sludge, genetically modified organisms, or ionizing radiation. Note: standards of organic farming vary.

P

Psyllium Husk - psyllium husks are portions of the seeds of the plant plantago. They are hygroscopic, which allows them to expand and become mucilaginous and be used as a natural firming or gelling agent.

Q

Quinoa - Quinoa is an ancient grain that can be eaten sprouted and uncooked or cooked in a way similar to preparing rice.

R

Raw - raw refers to food that is uncooked (not heated above 115° Fahrenheit /46° Celcius) and is in its natural state.

S

Sea Moss - sea moss, commonly called Irish moss or carrageen moss, is a species of red algae which grows abundantly along the rocky parts of the Atlantic coasts of Europe and North America, including the Caribbean.

Sea Salt (Celtic) - sea salt is salt harvested from the evaporation of seawater.

Soak/Soaked - soak or soaked refers to making or allowing food (primarily nuts and seeds) to become thoroughly wet by immersing it in liquid. By soaking nuts and seeds the enzyme inhibitors are removed and they become more digestible and nutrient-rich (see guide on page 119).

Spiralizer - a machine used in the kitchen for cutting vegetables very thinly into noodle-like shapes.

Sprout/Sprouted - sprout/sprouted refers primarily to nuts/seeds/grains that have been germinated through the process of soaking for a certain length of time then drained (and sometimes dehydrated   see guide on page 119).

T, U

Teflex Sheet/Teflex - a teflex sheet is a non-stick dehydrator sheet.

V

Vanilla Bean Paste — vanilla bean paste is made by infusing vanilla beans into a thick syrup made with sugar (raw date sugar) and water.

W, X, Y, & Z

Wakame - wakame is a highly nutritious seaweed (sea vegetable) often served in soups and salads.

Soaking & Sprouting Guide

Variety	Measure, Pre Soak (Dry)	Measure, Post Soak	Soaking Time	Sprouting/ Germination Time
Almonds	1 cup	1 and 1/2 cups	12 hours	0 hours
Brazil Nuts	1 cup	1 and 1/2 cups	6 hours	0 hours
Butternut Squash Seeds	1/4 cup	1/3 cup	8 hours	0 hours
Hazelnuts	1 cup	1 and 1/2 cups	6 hours	0 hours
Pecans	1 cup	1 and 1/2 cups	6 hours	0 hours
Walnuts	1 cup	1 and 1/2 cups	6 hours	0 hours
Chickpeas	1 cup	1 and 1/2 cups	12 hours	3 days
Amaranth	1 cup	3 cups	6 hours	24 hours
Quinoa	1 cup	1 and 1/2 cups	6 hours	3 days
Teff	1/2 cup	3/4 cup	3 hours	0
Wild Rice	2 cups	4 cups	12 hours	0

Note: Soaking/sprouting time may vary with environmental conditions.

Index

A
absorb 6
alkaline 3
almonds 4

B
breakfast 5
budget 4

C
carob 9, 28, 36, 37, 40
change 1
committed 1
consume 3
creative 2
culinary 2
curiosity 1, 2

D
dehydrator 4, 5
delicious 7, 1, 2, 5
depleted 2
diet 1, 2, 3, 4
dinner 5

E
encourage 6
energetic 2
experience 1, 2, 6
experiment 4

F
failure 5
food 1, 2, 3, 4, 5

G
fortify 6
fortifying 1
foundation 7, 1
fruits 3, 4

G
genetically modified organism 3
grateful 3, 1
gratitude 2
grocery 4, 6

H
habits 4
health 7, 1
healthier 7
herbs 3
holistic 7

I
ingredients 4
intelligence 5

J
journey 5, 1
juicer 4

K
kind 3, 4, 5

L
leafy greens 3, 4
life 7, 1, 2, 3, 4, 5

lifestyle 7, 1
love 3, 7, 1, 2, 5

M

mental health.. 2
milk 8, 13, 14
modalities... 2

N

non-gmo 3
non-hybrid 3
nourishing 7
nurturing.. 1
nutritious 7
nuts.. 3

P

palate 4
personal journey 1
pescatarian... 3
physical 2
plant-based 3, 4
practices 1
prepare 5
preparing... 2, 4, 5
process 1, 3
profound 1

Q

quinoa 3

R

raw 2, 7, 1, 2, 3, 4, 5, 6, 117, 118
recipes 2, 7, 2, 5

S

SAD 2, 4, 5, 6
seeds 3
self-esteem 1
self-love 1
self-loving 7
shake 9, 11, 15
simple 7, 1, 2
smoothie 5
soy 3
spiritually 6
Standard American Diet 2, 4
starch 3
stress relief 2
substantial.. 5
supportive 1

T

transitioning 2

U

universe 1, 2

V

vegan.. 2, 7, 1, 2, 3, 4, 5, 6
vegetarian 3

W

wellness 1, 2

Y

yoga 1, 2

Z

zero 7, 128

Special Thanks to the Teams at:

Align Your Health® Publishing House

AYH Live Foods Test Kitchens

John R. Winters Jr. Independent Editing

Numbers & Media, LLC.

SYSWC Marketing & Business Development, Inc.

TableTop™ Photography, Inc.

Thank you for your support, business advice, and guidance which contributed to the success of this book.

Copyright © 2016 by Align Your Health® Publishing House.
All Rights Reserved, including the right to reproduce this book and/or its contents in any form.

Printed in the United States of America

SYSWC Marketing and Business Development, Inc.
Align Your Health® Publishing House
5 Awbury Road
Philadelphia, Pennsylvania 19138
www.ayhlife.com

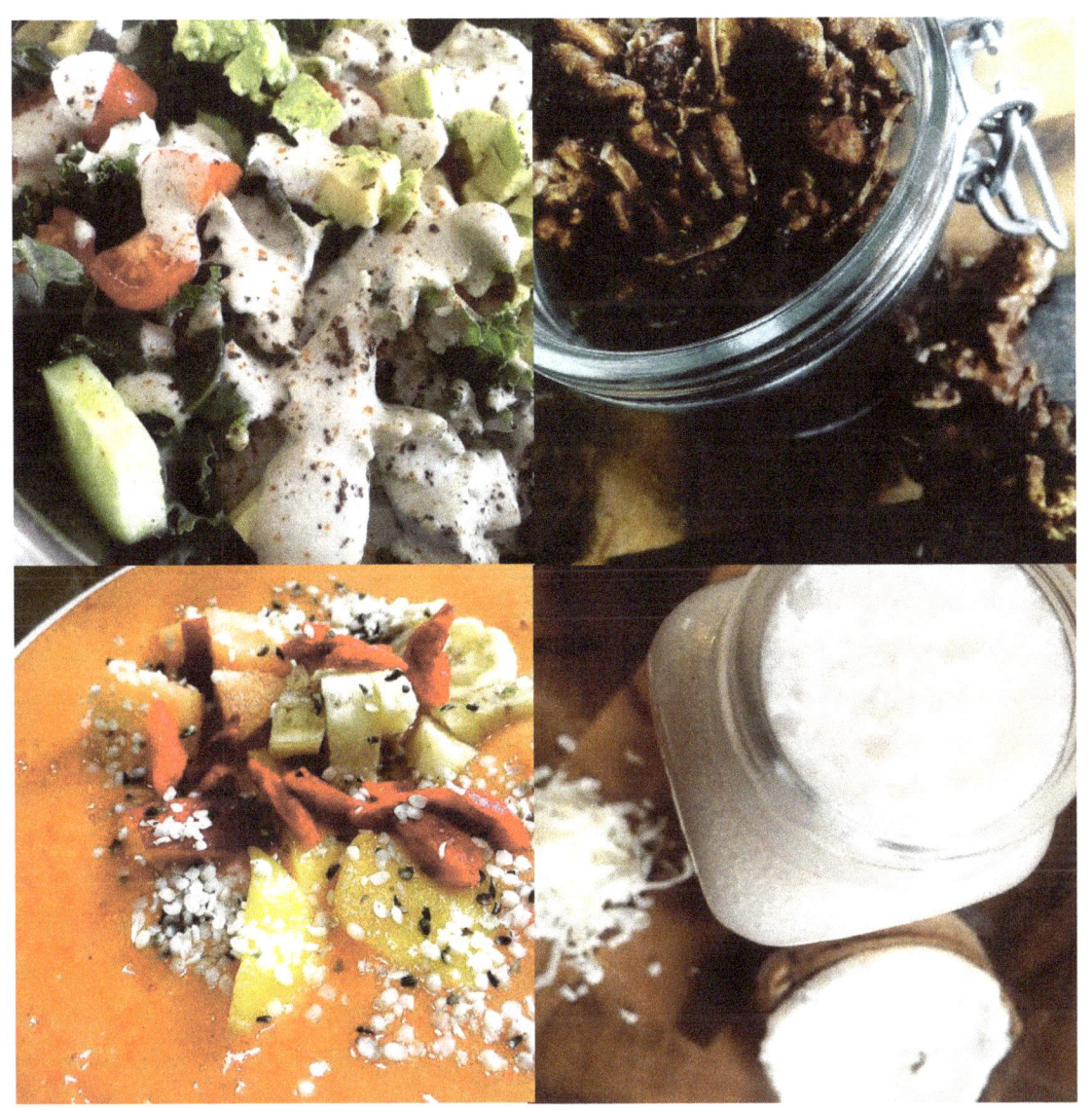

eat!

easy everyday raw vegan recipes!

K.L. Strayhorn

www.ingramcontent.com/pod-product-compliance
Lightning Source LLC
Chambersburg PA
CBHW061929290426
44113CB00024B/2849